THE **4** × **4** DIET

THE **4** × **4** DIET

---

4 Key Foods,

4-Minute Workouts,

Four Weeks to the Body You Want

Erin Oprea

Foreword by Carrie Underwood

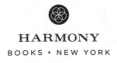

HARMONY

BOOKS • NEW YORK

Copyright © 2016 by Erin Oprea
Foreword copyright © 2016 by Carrie Underwood

Published in the United States by Harmony Books, an imprint
of the Crown Publishing Group, a division of Penguin Random
House LLC, New York.
www.crownpublishing.com

Harmony Books is a registered trademark, and the Circle
colophon is a trademark of Penguin Random House LLC.

Library of Congress Cataloging-in-Publication Data
Oprea, Erin.
    The 4 x 4 diet / Erin Oprea. —First edition.
        pages cm
1. Weight loss. 2. Reducing exercise. 3. Reducing diets—Recipes.
I. Title. II. Title: Four by four diet.
    RM222.2.O67 2016
    613.2′5—dc23
                                                2015030824
ISBN 978-1-101-90308-7
eBook ISBN 978-1-101-90309-4

PRINTED IN THE UNITED STATES OF AMERICA

Book design by Elizabeth Rendfleisch
Photographs by Carla Lynn Photography
Jacket design by Christopher Brand

10 9 8 7 6 5 4 3 2 1

First Edition

This book is dedicated to my mother, Ann.

For more years than is fair she has been my sounding board.

When I need advice, encouragement, a taste-tester, an honest eye,

someone to talk me off a ledge, and even someone to help me leap,

she has never flinched. I wrote a book, Mom. Did you see that coming?

This, in honor of you.

CONTENTS

PART 3: Getting Lean

PART 4: The 4 × 4 Diet

ACKNOWLEDGMENTS

Thank you!

Katy Lindenmuth—TeamBook captain, certified bada$$ writer and friend. Thank you for keeping your cool around me not keeping mine. Oh, and for helping me with the entire book!

Ann Stewart—Mom, you've been amazing for me.

Sean—Thank you for your endless love and support throughout this process. I couldn't have done it without your creativity, your dedication, and most importantly your patience. I love you!

Hunter and Hayden—I love you both so much. Thank you for being patient (mostly) with me during all my long workdays.

Carla Lynn—Your attention to detail and support of my vision did not go unnoticed.

My clients—Thank you for all your support. You hear about my whole life and hold no judgment, only encouragement. You would be surprised to know how much I value your opinions. Even if you think I'm cruel and unusual during our workouts.

Courtney Cain—Girl, you've seen my crazy. Good thing I've seen yours too. Thank you for everything.

Randy Word—Did you know that you were the one that sparked this whole idea? Probably not, you're very reserved. Thank you, Randy.

Sarah and Michael—Thank you both for grounding me and for your willingness to meet up at the drop of a hat. Having friends that you can count on to be exactly what you need, where you need them, and who have a complete willingness to share appetizers is invaluable.

FOREWORD

It's my personal belief that people take special care of the things that they love. Whether it's a car that's constantly being cleaned and waxed, a dream house that took years to save up for, or even a pair of shoes or a handbag by an *it* designer that makes every night out feel special. The bottom line is: If you love it, you want to keep it in pristine condition so it'll last forever. If we treat the things that we love like they're made of gold, why don't we treat our bodies like the amazing, powerful gifts that they are? It seems like, in today's world, we are constantly being told to love ourselves and to love our bodies. Of course we should! Our bodies can do incredible things! So why do we take them for granted? Why do we fill our bodies with food and drink that will harm them? Why don't we fuel them right, push them to their limits, make them strong, and make the most of what they can do? It took me asking these questions of myself to make a change in my own life. Once I realized that I did, in fact, love my body and myself, I decided that I was going to treat myself like the awesome person that I am with this one body that I have! I began with drinking more water, reading food labels, and questioning what was in the foods that I ate. I also decided to start working out more. And, soon after, that is when I met Erin Oprea.

I've had the pleasure of working with Erin for many years now and her approach to food, fitness, and overall health has not only been effective, but it's practical as well. Erin has taught me a lot about physical fitness and has helped me move from "dieting" to maintaining a consistent healthy lifestyle. The 4 × 4 Diet is a philosophy that anyone can implement into their daily lives in order to change the way they think about what they put into their bodies. It's not a diet . . . it's a lifestyle. Because if you treat your body like you love it, it will love you back!

Good luck on your journey! May your body reach its full potential, and may you reap all the benefits that treating yourself well can bring!

Carrie Underwood

INTRODUCTION

When I started my personal training career twenty years ago, never in my wildest dreams did I think I would someday be working with celebrities like Carrie Underwood, Jennifer Nettles, and Lee Ann Womack. But by developing and implementing my proven training method, the 4 × 4 Diet, I've helped my clients sculpt and maintain the toned physiques they've become famous for.

Sounds glamorous, right? Well, not exactly—a more apt description would be "constant, organized chaos." My workday begins at 3:30 a.m. and consists of back-to-back clients until dinnertime. I essentially live out of my car during the day, so I keep it stocked with all the meals, snacks, water, and workout equipment I may need. After a quick, healthy dinner at home, my whole family heads out the door for our evening activities— either my two sons have a couple of hours of soccer practice or my husband and I have a soccer game of our own. By the time we get back home, it's time for bed so I can wake up early and be rested enough to do it all over again . . . even on weekends.

My career is extremely demanding and rewarding, in equal parts, and it keeps me busy nearly every single minute of the day. I can't imagine spending my life doing anything else, but it was an interesting road that got me here. Before I began prepping clients for red-carpet events and video shoots, I was embedded deep in an active war zone in Iraq. (Twice.) And while I've always been into exercise, it took the sudden death of my father to realize how much nutrition plays a role in overall health, too. These and other personal experiences have led me to dedicate my life to health and fitness—specifically, the **clean and lean lifestyle**, which is the foundation of my **4 × 4 Diet**.

And a curiosity about the 4 × 4 Diet is the reason you picked up this book, right? Maybe the title jumped out at you. Maybe you're a Carrie Underwood fan and want to follow in her extremely toned footsteps. Or maybe you buy every single fitness book that comes out in the hopes that it will be the one that *finally* works for you. Regardless of what led you to be reading these pages right now, my message to you is the same: get ready to embrace four new clean eating habits, master the four-minute workout that my clients absolutely love, and see some incredible changes to your body within a month of starting the program.

Let's get to it—on the count of four.

PART 1

THE CLEAN AND LEAN LIFESTYLE

CHAPTER 1

The Road to Living Clean and Lean

I grew up in Sacramento, San Diego, and then Nashville, playing sports like soccer and swimming all along the way. I was constantly active starting at a young age, thanks in large part to my dad—he's the one who introduced me to soccer, and he later coached my high school team. (I still play competitively, and I even met my husband on the soccer field. He's also a personal trainer and fellow fitness freak.) My dad was always moving, whether it was tackling a 150-mile bike ride or opting for the stairs over the elevator. Our lifestyle wasn't simply about being athletic—it was about being active.

As a teenager, I was eager to finish high school. I knew I wanted to share my passion for fitness with all kinds of people, so I graduated at sixteen and became a certified trainer within two years. By this point, I had honed the "lean" part of my clean and lean philosophy: **The more you move, the more you stay lean.** It was simple and clearly effective—all anyone had to do was look at my dad's and my trim physiques, which we attributed to our active lifestyle. I preached this motto often.

But I was also eager to keep challenging myself physically. So when I was twenty, I enlisted in the Marines, and I served two tours in Iraq between 2003 and 2005. The day before I was scheduled to leave for my second deployment, a group of friends and family gathered at my parents' house for a going-away cookout. At one point, my dad walked over to my mom and told her that his chest hurt. The two of them went inside, and she turned around to get something for him—and that's when he suddenly fell over and died. Instantly. The doctors later told us that he was dead before he even hit the ground. Within three minutes, he went from feeling ill to suffering a fatal heart attack.

My dad was just fifty-two when he passed away. He had been trim and strong his whole life—he'd *thrived* on being physically active—and he'd never had any major health issues. So how did this happen? The answer was crushing: for more than five decades, he had eaten whatever he wanted, whenever he wanted. He'd never been told to watch his diet, to eat certain foods, and to avoid certain others. For me, it was the hardest way to learn that being thin doesn't necessarily mean being healthy.

My father's sudden death changed everything for me. After I took ten days of military emergency leave, duty called. It was heartbreaking to leave my family—especially my mom—when the pain was still so fresh, but I had to follow through on my commitment and return to Iraq.

Upon arriving, I threw myself into work. This was 2004, and Fallujah had been shut down. When Iraqi citizens were finally being let back in the city, every individual had to be searched. Men weren't allowed to physically touch the women, so the Marines' first-ever all-female platoon was created—and my superiors appointed me as the sergeant to train and lead that search force. One of my main duties was to look for suicide bombers, contraband, and guns at various checkpoints around Fallujah. It was *intense*—and I loved every minute of it. I actually tried to extend my stay, but my commanding officer made me come home.

After returning to Nashville, I finally started to process my dad's death. My way of doing this was by learning everything I could about food and how it affects your body. I took nutrition seminars, experimented endlessly with recipes, and eventually became certified as a nutrition coach. One of my biggest revelations was that I began to see food as fuel for your body—not as a reward or as a hobby—and I set out to discover the most efficient ways to use it. The answer, in short, is to maintain a diet with as many whole foods and as few processed foods as possible. Fresh fruits and vegetables, lean meats, legumes, nuts—*these* are what your body should be running on. My findings ultimately became the "clean" part of my clean and lean philosophy.

Over the next few years, I began training elite clients and instilling in them the virtues of being clean *and* lean—not just one or the other. In my own kitchen, I continued to experiment with all kinds of recipes and ingredients, working toward the cleanest and best-tasting diet possible. The process is ever-evolving, but I've pinned down four key eating habits: cutting out starches at night and cutting back on your sugar, sodium, and alcohol intake. Practicing all four of these habits regularly has produced the most dramatic effects on my own body and my clients' bodies. Meanwhile, I also discovered an innovative four-minute workout called tabata that shocked me with its (science-backed) effectiveness.

Grabbing onto the "4" element of each discovery, I developed the 4 × 4 Diet. The combination of these four clean eating habits and four-minute workouts has been a game-changer for me as well as for my clients, who span just about every age, body type, and fitness level. Listen, I am *always* excited to eat healthy and try new exercises. It's my job, it's my passion, and it's also my lifestyle. But the 4 × 4 Diet has gotten my clients—people who have struggled with weight loss and motivation for years—to be excited to clean up their diet and work out. And now I want to share it with you.

CHAPTER 2

What Is Clean and Lean?

The 4 × 4 Diet was built on a simple two-part philosophy that I've been practicing for over a decade: **Eat clean and get lean.** It's the key to becoming the healthiest you possible—and each part is equally important. Once you understand what it is and how it works, you can use the clean and lean philosophy to unlock the power of the 4 × 4 Diet.

So where did the name come from? For each of the two components, the magic number is—you guessed it—4: **In my program, eating clean consists of four key habits, and getting lean consists of a four-minute workout called tabata.** In this book, I'll explain how I came to these conclusions and show you how to gradually incorporate both parts into your daily life through the four-week program that I created. If you stick with it, within a month you can expect to see and feel results that include the following:

- increased muscle definition in your arms, legs, and stomach
- reduced bloating and puffiness from your cheeks to your toes
- improved cardiovascular endurance
- the breaking of sugar and sodium addictions you may have been battling your whole life (without even realizing it!)

I do want to forewarn you that this book is not simply pointers on healthy eating and photos of workout moves. The 4 × 4

Diet goes much deeper than that—it involves learning the "why" behind the "what": *why* you're making a certain sauce instead of buying it in a jar; *why* you're pushing yourself as hard as you can during those four-minute tabata exercises; *why* you're avoiding certain foods before dinner; *why* you're repeating a series of one-legged squats. Over the next several chapters, I'll be giving you the condensed version of everything I've learned over the years—and, luckily for you, I'm cutting out all the dead ends and hypotheses that didn't pan out for me. It's still a ton of information, but I'm presenting it in a way that is easy to follow and digest. So don't get overwhelmed or feel like there's just too much to learn. Knowledge is power, after all, and it's what you need to know to become your healthiest *you*. So let's dive in.

The Clean Philosophy

Eating clean boils down to one idea: consuming more whole foods, also known as "real" foods, unrefined foods, or unprocessed foods. Clean foods have had minimal interference between their origin (e.g., the tree or animal they came from) and their final destination (that'd be your mouth). If it comes in a bag, box, or can, it's probably processed.

Clean eating is a simple idea to understand but not *quite* as simple to commit to completely. In fact, it can be pretty darn complicated. That's because processed foods are everywhere you turn, from grocery store shelves to your favorite restaurant to the airport grab-and-go kiosk. It is shocking how many processed foods people consume without realizing it—in fact, one analysis estimates that highly processed foods make up more than 60 percent of the calories in the food that we buy. Even more shocking is the toll these common foods take on your body over time, whether it's adding on pounds, screwing with your metabolism, or paving the way for heart disease. (My father's sudden fatal heart attack is a tragic example of the worst outcome.)

Here's where the clean lifestyle fits into the 4 × 4 Diet: the first "4" refers to four specific clean eating habits that, when practiced

- It's not something you could find in nature, like on a tree, in the ocean, or in the ground.
- It comes in a box, bag, can, or other manufactured form of packaging.
- It has a noticeably long ingredients list.
- It contains additives, artificial flavorings, and/ or other chemicals, especially ones that are hard to pronounce.
- It contains vegetable or seed oil.
- It's not found on the perimeter of the grocery store.

regularly, can translate to weight loss and lowered risk of debilitating illnesses like heart disease, diabetes, and even cancer. They'll also steady out your blood sugar level, which in turn can increase your energy. And these habits can completely reinvigorate your mind and your overall mood by boosting production of a brain neurotransmitter called serotonin, which your body needs to maintain a certain level of in order to function properly. (It's no coincidence that most health nuts—myself included—are constantly chipper!) A clean lifestyle will upgrade you from head to toe and from inside out.

I've been practicing a clean diet for more than a decade now, ever since I threw myself into learning about nutrition back in 2005. I've also coached my clients into a clean eating lifestyle and watched their bodies transform day by day. These are the four habits that, when combined and practiced consistently, have produced the most striking results:

Cutting out starches at night
Cutting back on sugar
Cutting back on sodium
Cutting back on alcohol

As you can see, they're pretty straightforward. You may even occasionally practice a couple of these habits, like opting for the low-sodium version of your favorite soup or "detoxing" from booze for a couple weeks. But, as with clean eating as a whole, these are commitments that will take some getting used to—especially when all four are combined. With the 4 × 4 Diet, I'll show you how to effectively boost your metabolism and become a clean eating pro in just one month.

As you transition into a clean eating lifestyle, it's crucial to remember that you're not eliminating anything fully from your diet. You're not depriving yourself of a particular food. You're not swearing off pizza or wine for the rest of your life. Instead, you're retooling what you put into your body so that it can be used as efficiently as possible.

Getting Clean Starts Here

One of the healthiest things you can do for your body is also one of the easiest and cheapest: keep it hydrated. This is often the first lesson I go over with all of my clients, and that's for good reason. Water affects virtually every part of your body, inside and out. It flushes out toxins and carries essential nutrients into your cells. Your joints, spinal cord, and organs are all cushioned by fluid, and staying hydrated is vital to their well-being. Hydration kick-starts the breaking down of every piece of food that you put into your mouth—when you are unable to produce enough saliva, your body has to play catch-up while extracting the vital nutrients from your meals (plus it triggers that awful dry-mouth feeling). Finally, being hydrated becomes even more crucial when you're working out. In addition to transporting oxygen to your brain and to your muscles, allowing you to physically get up and move, water is promptly kicked out of your body via sweat. Clearly, water is a big deal to your body—the only thing it needs more of to function properly is oxygen.

Unfortunately, though, many people become dehydrated without realizing it, and over time either they get used to, fail to recognize, or simply ignore the symptoms. The primary symptom is obvious: if you're dehydrated, you'll feel thirsty. *Really* thirsty—to the point where your mouth becomes dry and sticky, like sandpaper. Another common symptom is noticeable fatigue or sluggishness. Less common symptoms include dizziness, heart palpitations, dark yellow urine, weakness, muscle cramps, overheating, dry skin, headaches, lightheadedness, and loss of skin elasticity. If you regularly find yourself with any of these symptoms and think it may be due to dehydration, start logging and increasing your H_2O intake. (And, of course, if the symptoms are severe—like if you're no longer urinating or you're having difficulty breathing—you'll want to see a doctor ASAP.)

Your skin may be able to tell you if you're dehydrated. Use two fingers to pinch the skin on the back of one hand, between where a watch would sit and where your fingers start. Pull the skin up about a half centimeter to one centimeter high and then release it. The skin should spring back to its normal position in less than a couple of seconds. If it takes longer than that, you could be dehydrated.

So how much water should you be drinking? According to the Institute of Medicine, women should have about nine glasses of water every day and men should have about thirteen—at a minimum. **My general rule is to drink half your body weight in ounces of water per day.** That means if you weigh 140 pounds, you'd shoot for 70 ounces, or just under 9 glasses. If you weigh 170 pounds, you'd shoot for 85 ounces, or about 10.5 glasses.

Of course, there's some fine print here. You need to drink more water before, during, and after every workout, since you'll be sweating it out. You also need to drink more water if you're eating salty foods, like marinades and packaged snacks, to counterbalance the deluge of sodium in your body. (You'll learn more about sodium's role in a clean diet—and how to limit your intake—in Chapter 4.) And you need to keep your surrounding environment in mind: hot and humid weather can make you sweat, and high altitudes can make you pee more. Both of these instances require extra hydration.

Here are some sneaky ways to drink more water:

- Keep a full glass or sports bottle of water on your nightstand so that it's the first thing you see when you wake up. (And make sure you actually drink it.)
- Carry a full bottle of water with you all day long.

- Keep track of your intake by refilling your bottle as soon as you drink it completely.
- Flavor your water with a tasty natural food, like a slice of lemon, lime, or orange or a small handful of berries . . .
- . . . Or infuse it with herbs like mint or lavender.
- Eat something hot or spicy so that you're practically diving across the table for a water refill.
- Eat water-based foods like spinach, watermelon, tomatoes, and grapes—they count toward your daily water intake, too.
- Drink one last big glass before bed while you're brushing your teeth.

The Lean Philosophy

Let's start by going over what "lean" is *not*: It's *not* a target number on a scale. It's *not* a specific number on the body mass index (BMI) table. It's *not* a single-digit number stitched into the waist of your jeans. These kinds of numbers aren't worth getting hung up on because they don't tell the whole story.

Here's what lean is: to get technical, it's having a low percentage of body fat compared to your percentage of lean mass. (Lean body mass includes everything that's not considered fat, like muscles and bones.) One of the most common tools used to measure body fat, the body mass index, uses your height and weight. But since the BMI method's reliability is increasingly under scrutiny (National Public Radio has actually called it "bogus!"), I rely on a non-numerical definition that is a combination of how you look and feel. **"Lean" means looking fit, with visible muscle tone and minimal excess body fat for your particular body type. "Lean" also means feeling strong and full of energy.**

Your body has a fixed number of muscle fibers—that amount generally caps when you hit puberty. So as an adult, you can't control how many muscles you have—but you can control their size. The bigger they get, the tighter and stronger your physique.

Have you ever heard someone being described as "skinny-fat"? These people are thin on the surface—appearing to be in good health—often due to good genetics, a great metabolism, or sheer luck. But they have very little muscle tone due to their lack of physical activity; it may even be a struggle for them to walk up a couple flights of stairs. And their body is often a mess on the inside—think high risk for diabetes, high blood pressure, and high cholesterol. So focus on building up muscle and not just getting rid of fat!

And that's what sets "lean" apart from common diet terms like "skinny" and "thin"—because getting lean is not about simply losing weight or reducing your waist size. If a thigh gap is all you're focusing on, you're missing the point. You actually *need* some muscle mass in order to have the strength to go about your daily life, especially when you're exercising regularly and torching the calories that you're consuming. (In fact, the more muscle you have, the more calories you burn even at rest.) If you're just skinny—skin and bones and very little developed muscle—not only will you struggle to complete tough workouts, but you also may end up injuring yourself.

Now that you know what "lean" is, you're probably wondering: *How do I make my body lean?* That may be the main reason you are reading this book. And now I'll let you in on my biggest fitness secret weapon—it's the second "4" in the 4 × 4 Diet. **The most effective kind of workout that I use is a form of high-intensity interval training called tabata. One tabata lasts just four minutes.**

One tabata is:
20 seconds of high-intensity moves,
then 10 seconds of rest,
repeated 8 times.

A four-minute workout that actually produces a lean, healthy body? I can't wait to show you exactly how it works—it's based on a landmark scientific study inspired by Japanese speed skaters. I also can't wait for you to try it yourself. But hold that thought until Chapter 9. Let's work our way there together.

Getting Lean Starts Here

Before you learn the four-minute workout—before you throw yourself into any kind of regular exercise, really—you need to build a strong foundation. Getting lean begins with embracing an active lifestyle and moving as much as possible as you go about your day. Studies have shown that the more sedentary you are, the higher your risk of diabetes, cardiovascular disease, and obesity. On the flip side, regular physical activity can boost your energy level, sleep quality, and overall mood. It also, of course, gets you closer to becoming—and staying—lean.

If you're starting from zero and currently leading a truly sedentary lifestyle, your regular physical activity shouldn't consist of full-on high-intensity workouts. (Those will come later!) But it *must* involve a healthy dose of low-impact activity—specifically, walking a certain number of steps every day. **If you're not already physically active, you should start by taking about 5,000 steps per day.** Just get up and walk, wherever and whenever you can. As you become accustomed to this increase in activity, walk an additional few hundred or thousand steps per day, working your way toward the ultimate goal: twice that amount.

Yup, **if you're already working out regularly, you should be taking 10,000 steps per day**—that's the equivalent of about five miles and what's recommended by the American Heart Association. It's also the goal I set for myself and almost all of my clients.

Ten thousand is a lot of steps to count in your head. The easiest way to keep track is by investing in a pedometer. From the electronics aisle to online retailers, today's available options run the gamut. Older models clip to your belt or shoe and usually have a few easy-to-use settings. These are great for the not-so-tech-savvy crowd as well as anyone who's not into devices with bells and whistles. Then there are newer bracelet-like varieties—this is the option many of my clients and I prefer—that offer additional functions like goal setting and calorie counting, are generally more durable, and can sync to your smartphone and computer. FitBit, Jawbone, and Garmin all offer solid fitness trackers.

While these tools' exact level of accuracy is a topic of debate,

I've found that wearing one regularly is extremely useful in terms of comparing your day-to-day activity. In that sense, they're undeniably self-motivating: just having one on your wrist or belt loop is a constant reminder that, quite literally, every step counts.

Walking itself is easy. Think about it: you've been doing it almost your entire life, so you've had decades of practice. Walking 10,000 steps every single day, on the other hand, is not as easy. I consider myself lucky because, starting at a young age, it was ingrained in me to constantly be moving—for me, it just feels weird to sit still for more than a few minutes at a time. But I know that's not always the case and that it's easy to get comfortable, especially if you spend a lot of time sitting at a desk for your job. (Again, I'm lucky that my job requires me to be running from place to place.) Whether you're new to exercise or already accustomed to being active, there are endless ways to work up to those 10,000 daily steps. A few of these may seem like common sense—but have you actually tried them?

Here are some sneaky ways to walk a little bit more every day:

- Get into a walking routine, whether it's three short walks every day or five long ones per week.
- Start taking your dog on longer walks—it'll improve your pet's health, too!
- Always take the steps instead of the elevator or escalator (or at least take them on the way down).
- Set an alarm on your computer or phone reminding you to get up and walk around every hour or two.
- Initiate a walking meeting at work, if weather (and your boss) permits.
- Every time you run outside to the mailbox or to take out the trash, take a loop around the block. (And please don't *drive* to your mailbox!)
- Hop off the subway or bus one or two stops early.
- At the office, use the bathroom and/or kitchen one floor above or below yours.

- Whenever possible, deliver messages in person rather than by phone or e-mail (like to your coworker or your friend who lives a few streets over).
- March in place while doing standstill tasks like brushing your teeth, drying your hair, or talking on the phone.
- Pace the room anytime you're stuck waiting for an appointment or lap the parking lot while your kids finish up with practice.
- Set up your alarm clock a few rooms away to add extra steps before you're even fully awake.
- Park farther away than usual from your office or the grocery store (or park in your assigned spot and lap the building before heading inside).
- Walk around your airport gate if you arrive early for your flight or if it's delayed—some airports have even started posting the mileage between gates, concourses, and terminals.
- Whenever you're shopping, lap the perimeter of the store and then walk up and down every aisle.
- The point is to get into the habit of moving as much as you can, so get creative with it! Whatever you do, wherever you go, always be thinking about how you can walk just a little bit more than you did yesterday.

The 4 × 4 Diet

Over the past ten years, through my own trial and error as well as through watching my clients overcome serious health hurdles, I've used the clean and lean philosophy to develop the 4 × 4 Diet. The program is one part nutrition, one part fitness—and by now, you know the basics. The rest? I explain it all over the following chapters.

In Part 2, I break down the first "4" of the 4 × 4 Diet: the four clean eating habits that I mentioned above. I'll tell you why and how to cut out starches at night and cut down on sugar, sodium, and alcohol—once you realize how much they can damage your body, you'll be even more motivated to scale back. I'm also excited to share with you the specific techniques I use to stay on top of my nutrition game—that includes a bunch of all-star ingredients, a few handy kitchen tools, simple substitutions for certain not-so-good-for-you foods, and, of course, loads of delicious recipes for every type of meal.

In Part 3, I'll introduce you to the second "4" of the 4 × 4 Diet: the tabata workout. Through detailed instructions and photos, I'll show you thirty of these four-minute exercises, in Beginner, Intermediate, and Advanced levels. Once you nail those, you can mix and match them, modify them to make them easier or harder, and create entirely new tabatas altogether to form a complete, customized workout that you love. I'll also arm you with some other important workout tools: how to warm up and cool down as well as the pieces of equipment that I use myself and with my clients. We don't use many, but the ones we do really pack a punch.

Finally, in Part 4, I'll show you how to combine the four clean eating habits and the four-minute tabata workouts. Together, they form the 4 × 4 Diet, and you'll roll out all the elements over the course of one month, gradually incorporating them into your lifestyle. There's no single "correct" way to do this—it depends on your current fitness level and diet regimen. To guide you along, I've put together clean and lean objectives for each week, the results you can expect as you go along, and sample workout and eating plans.

You'll start to see and feel changes within a week. With this kind of regular exercise, your arms and legs will gain muscle definition—not just because your muscle fibers have expanded, but because you're simultaneously reducing the layer of fat covering them and they can now actually be seen. (This happens most noticeably when you begin to reduce the amount of bloat-causing sodium in your diet.) And a huge perk of the four-minute workouts is that, due to their bursts of intensity, as you progress, they can improve your endurance better than a regular workout can.

As incredible as these changes are, they're only the beginning. The real reward happens by *maintaining* this healthy lifestyle, because those results will keep evolving long after the thirty days are up. And that should be your ultimate goal: to turn these new habits into your new normal.

As the weeks, months, and years go on, you'll continue to look and be even stronger. You'll feel cleaner and look leaner. You'll forget what it was like to rely on pasta dishes for dinner or to hole up in your office all day without getting up for a walk. **I know the 4 × 4 Diet works because I've seen the results in myself and in my clients.** They're leaner, stronger, and the healthiest possible version of themselves. Are you ready to join them?

CHAPTER 3

Overcoming Excuses

When it comes to not being able to work out and eat well, I've heard every excuse imaginable. I've been doing this for over twenty years, after all. Plus, I train a lot of people who are creative for a living—they can come up with some pretty interesting arguments.

If you are reading this book, there's a good chance that you, too, are guilty of playing the blame game to avoid a workout or a steady healthy diet. Allow me to use this chapter to explain why that's a bad idea.

THE MOST COMMON EXCUSES FOR NOT WORKING OUT

WORKOUT EXCUSE #1: "I'm too busy."

Ah, the classic excuse. Trust me, I get it—when you have kids to shuttle around, meetings or exams to prep for, and meals to cook at home, exercise is usually what gets shoved to the bottom of the to-do list. Sometimes you may fantasize about where you'll squeeze it into your schedule (how many times have you sworn that you'll make the 6 a.m. kickboxing class or lunch-hour boot camp?). Other times you may panic just *thinking* about the amount of time it takes out of your day: there's the drive or walk to the gym, the actual hourlong workout, the commute home, the shower. . . . That could easily suck almost two hours out of your day. It would be great to have that much free time, but how many of us actually do?

Here's the trick: you just *think* you're too busy for a solid workout. **Not every workout has to last an hour or take place at the gym. In fact, often the best ones do neither.** The four-minute tabata workouts I show you in Chapter 12 are ideal for people exactly like you and make up the bulk of my training sessions and my own workouts. While you're mastering the tabata style, though, there are plenty of other ways to work other kinds of exercise into a jam-packed schedule.

Here are some of my favorite multitasking fitness tricks:

- **Stash a jump rope in your car** and bust it out during downtime at your kids' sports practice. (You may inspire other parents to do the same.)
- **Make date night more active.** My husband and I once took weekly hip-hop classes instead of going out for dinner. It was a hilarious way to burn calories and spend time together. (It's on YouTube—we have no shame.)
- **Make family time more active, too.** You're more likely to find my kids and me running a community 5K than at the movie theater.
- **Take a brisk walk** while making phone calls, whether they're business-related or to catch up with an old friend.
- **Engage your body** while sitting at your desk. I'm actually doing butt squeezes as I type this.

WORKOUT EXCUSE #2: "I'm injured" or "I'm sick."

Many of my clients suffer from the occasional injury or illness—a sore back, mild shoulder pain, an unfortunately timed cold. Personally, I've had two knee surgeries and sporadic wrist issues. If you're ailing, despite your immediate instincts, you *can* still burn calories and continue to tone up. In fact, by not working out as you wait to recover, you actually could be doing your body more harm than good. **Staying active can help you bounce back more quickly from an injury.** A great example of this is a married couple I train who are in their seventies. They took a nasty tumble together off a curb last year—they were holding hands, and when she went down, he followed. The wife was more seriously injured: she broke her hip. But they both recovered ahead of schedule. Their doctor told them this was because of the strength they'd built up from our twice-weekly training sessions.

There are lots of ways you can safely keep moving while taking care of what hurts. I've put together a list of regular exercises you can do when one or more body parts are out of commission. Turn to page 197 to learn how to work around these injuries and ailments:

- A sore knee or ankle
- A sore back
- A sore shoulder
- A sore wrist or elbow
- A cold or allergies
- Bunions
- A stomachache or menstrual cramps
- Constipation
- Exhaustion
- Lightheadedness

WORKOUT EXCUSE #3: "I'm so out of shape that there's no point."

This one breaks my heart: some people truly believe it's hopeless for them to work out. They've tried it in the past, but they didn't lose weight. Or they didn't lose *enough* weight. Or they did lose weight, but then they gained it back. For these people, I start by echoing what I tell clients who say they're too tired to work out: just get moving, no matter how you do it—any kind of physical activity is better than remaining sedentary. **Sitting stirs more laziness, and moving stirs more energy.**

But I also tell them something else. This is where the clean lifestyle comes roaring back into play. I can guarantee that the people who say exercising "didn't work" for them weren't eating smartly. They likely were partaking in fad diets—which by design are not sustainable—and then resorting back to their old, unhealthy food habits. These are yo-yo dieters, meaning they are super-restrictive for two weeks or two months, and when the designated amount of time is up—or when they quit early out of frustration—they gain back the weight they lost, and sometimes a little extra.

That whole approach doesn't work because it's wrong. The 4 × 4 Diet is not about obliterating carbs or gluten from your diet for thirty days. It's not about drinking lemon water for a week. It's not about losing ten pounds before the weekend. It's about developing four specific food habits and learning why they lead to a healthy lifestyle. Paired with regular exercise, that leads to a better you. So get moving.

THE MOST COMMON EXCUSES FOR NOT EATING WELL

DIET EXCUSE #1: "I'm too busy."

Just as you *thought* you were too busy to work out regularly, you just *think* you don't have enough time to maintain a healthy diet. While there's no four-minute trick for producing a healthy, well-balanced meal, there are tons of ways to streamline the process of shopping for, prepping, and cooking your food. My family has developed a strategy called Prep Day (page 70), which is a designated time every week when we knock out as much food-related prep as humanly possible to get us through the next seven days. We'll do things such as sautéing snack nuts and baking chicken and then store them until they're ready to be eaten. Knocking out those little tasks all at once saves so much time and makes it less tempting to grab something unhealthy in the days ahead.

DIET EXCUSE #2: "Healthy food doesn't taste good."

I hear this excuse from people ages five to seventy-five. And I've found that most of the time, they haven't actually tried the foods they're protesting. So that's your first step: taste-test foods that you swear you don't like—whether it's lima beans, flounder, or soy milk—but can't remember exactly why.

The next trick is to change up how you're preparing the foods, thus altering their taste. Whether it's through a method like sautéing or a seasoning like rosemary, practically any food can be tweaked into a tastier state. A great example: maybe you don't like raw beets, but have you tried roasting them? Pop them in the oven and they become sweeter and softer.

Finally, if you *still* don't like the taste of a particular healthy food, just give it a few weeks or months. Your taste buds can actually adapt to certain foods—you'll see this in effect when you start to limit your sugar and sodium intake. Some sugary treats will become almost unbearably sweet, and salty foods you used to enjoy may leave you guzzling water. Those are signs that your clean diet is working its magic.

DIET EXCUSE #3: "I deserve a treat for my hard work."

I'm not a fan of a reward system that's based on this philosophy: "I worked out hard today, so now I can eat this junk food." Realistically, you probably didn't burn enough calories during that workout to make up for a huge bowl of pasta or pile of greasy fries. So all that hard work just went to waste. If you reward yourself with unhealthy food every time you work out, you'll *never* lose weight.

Here's some great news, though: "cheating" is allowed. **It's important to let yourself indulge in a craving once or twice a week— and not feel bad about it.** Eat or drink what you've been *really* missing so that you don't feel like you're depriving yourself. Whether it's loaded nachos or an extra glass of red wine, make sure you pause and enjoy it—and then get right back on track with your next meal and workout.

For my family, we allow ourselves one not-so-good dinner per week—we usually order a thin-crust pizza with pepperoni and bacon; that way, no one even has to lift a finger to prepare it. Just make sure you do it in moderation! One time, my client ate five donuts as a birthday "treat" and immediately got a massive stomachache because she hadn't eaten them in years. She felt so horrible that I guarantee she'll never do it again.

The smartest way to indulge is by planning it ahead of time—that could even mean scheduling it on your calendar. Say you have a work luncheon, a family member's birthday dinner, and an outing with friends all in one week. Decide which of those occasions you'll have your cheat meal at and then, just as importantly, map out how you'll stay true to your healthy ways during the others. (This tactic also works when it comes to getting into the habit of limiting your weekly alcohol intake, which we'll talk about on page 48.)

My clients lie to me all the time about how well they've been eating—I can always tell. I've found that when they finally do start cleaning up their diet, they feel, look, and act healthier. They smile more and receive more compliments. They're stunned by how much their diet truly affects their life and by what it's like to feel "normal." The lesson here? Be honest with yourself and what you're actually eating, because your body knows— and shows—the truth.

But let's be clear: don't view these meals as a reward for "being good all week"—on the contrary, you're rewarding yourself when you're fueling it with healthy food. Giving in to the occasional craving is okay simply because nobody's perfect.

PART 2

EATING CLEAN

CHAPTER 4

The 4 Clean Eating Habits

I never set out to create a four-week diet program. Or a diet program of any kind, really, especially one for the masses. For years, I was simply focused on eating as cleanly as possible—keeping myself and my family happy and healthy—and then relaying that information to my clients whenever they asked for guidance.

As several of my celebrity clients started becoming more and more well known for their toned figures (in addition to their day jobs), I found myself being approached by magazine editors who were excited to cite me as a fitness and nutrition expert. I began writing weekly blogs and articles for outlets online and in print, talking about the importance of hydration and demonstrating all kinds of exercise moves. I was reaching a whole new audience.

People I'd never met began asking me for diet tips, and their questions were usually along the lines of "What foods should I eat/not eat to lose weight?" or "What am I doing wrong?" My answer, always, was to eat a clean diet consisting of five daily meals: breakfast, midmorning snack, lunch, afternoon snack, and dinner. Then they'd ask where to start, since clean eating is such a broad topic. Without realizing it, my answer to that question was always the same, too. One day, something clicked—my clean eating philosophy has four main tenets that are easy to remember and to follow:

Cut out starches at night.

Cut back on sugar.

Cut back on sodium.

Cut back on alcohol.

The idea is really that simple. Once I had that epiphany—that the idea of clean eating had four distinct components—I knew I had to share it. I didn't want to call these four clean eating components *rules*—that's such an intimidating word. Rules are hard-and-fast regulations that you must follow to a T; if not, you'll get in trouble or be considered a failure. (That's no fun.) I didn't want to call them clean eating *tips*, either, because they're more than just handy tricks to bust out when you want to drop a few pounds for a big event. They're quite the opposite, actually—I've been practicing them for about ten years, and by now they're second nature.

And that's exactly why I decided to call them *habits*: they're behavior patterns acquired by frequent repetition. You do them so much that eventually you do them without thinking. That's the ideal clean lifestyle.

The 4 × 4 Diet is not a short-term solution. It's designed to give you four weeks to incorporate four clean eating habits into your life—and then the "diet" we started together becomes your healthy lifestyle. It's sustainable because these habits don't eliminate anything from your diet—rather, they're about consuming the proper amounts, at the time of day when your body will best use them.

The 4 × 4 Diet is a whole new lifestyle, especially when it comes to food. You'll likely be changing at least one part of every single meal you eat—that's a huge commitment. You'll constantly be faced with salty, sugary temptations. And you'll be incredibly tempted to give in, especially before you start seeing and feeling any results. So don't forget that a guilt-free indulgence—aka a cheat meal—once or twice a week is always allowed. After all, just as one good meal does not make you a healthy person, one bad meal does not ruin your diet. If you practice the four clean eating habits together, and consistently, throughout the rest of the week, what will emerge is the healthiest, happiest version of you.

CLEAN HABIT #1: Cut Out Starches at Night

The bad news: no more starchy foods, like pasta and potatoes, for dinner. The good news: you still get to enjoy them earlier in the day. Not a bad compromise when it means a leaner, cleaner you, right?

What you need to know about starches and your body

Starches are also known as complex carbohydrates because they're made of three or more sugar molecules that are strung together like a necklace or branched like a coil. For consistency's—and brevity's—sake throughout this book, I refer to them as starches. But they're the exact same thing.

Here's a sentence you probably didn't expect to find in a book about nutrition: **Carbs are fantastic**. They've been demonized for their caloric content in certain health circles and fad diet books—but they're just a little misunderstood, that's all. So let's get to know them and what they're capable of.

There are three kinds of carbohydrates: sugar, starch, and fiber. Two of those kinds, sugars and starches, serve as your body's main energy source. (Meanwhile, fiber has its own agenda that's full of important tasks like regulating bowel movements and controlling blood sugar.) This is why breakfast is considered the most important meal of the day and usually involves carbs like cereal, potatoes, and/or some form of bread. You're stocking up on energy to get you through whatever the day ahead holds. Adding to their appeal is that lots of carbs taste absolutely *delicious*— think pancakes, spaghetti, and my personal favorite, oatmeal.

See, what did I tell you? Carbs are pretty impressive.

But there's more to the story. A few years ago, I started really thinking about starches and their role as an energy source. In simple terms, here's what happens: after entering your body, starches are quickly broken down into molecules and get a cool new name: glucose. The glucose then enters your bloodstream and is distributed to every cell in your body. Your cells use up that glucose as energy. All of this happens rapidly after you swallow your food, which is why starches are considered a short-term energy source. That explains why you usually need to refuel at lunch in order to get through the afternoon without succumbing to the nap gods. (In case you were wondering, long-term energy sources include fats and protein, since they're not as easy for your body to break down.)

Starches are part of a pretty reliable system: input food, output energy. And if you don't use up that glucose for some reason, your cells can tuck away a small amount of it in your muscles and liver and then draw on it when you need a shot of energy (in storage form, by the way, it's called glycogen). But your body can only store a certain amount of glucose. What happens to the excess? It's stored as fat.

Remember how I was talking about how delicious carbs, especially starches, can be? Well, keep in mind that no potato or piece of bread is so tasty that it can't wait until the next morning to be eaten—and subsequently used up by your body.

And there's the catch—when you eat carbs later in the day, you usually aren't exerting much of that energy afterward. You're winding down from a day on your feet, lounging on the couch, helping the kids with homework, or catching up on a book. **Because you're not burning as many calories, your body is more likely to convert those carbs into fat.**

The 4 × 4 solution: **Fuel up your body with high-quality starches in the morning and afternoon, when you're the most active.** Go about your day, working toward your 10,000 steps, using them as your fuel. Then, in mid- to late afternoon, halt your starch intake—a good cutoff time is around 3 or 4 p.m. That means nothing starchy will be in your afternoon snack, dinner, dessert, or postdinner snack.

How to tell if a food is high in starch

- For processed and packaged foods, identifying starches is often as easy as reading the label. Starchy foods contain ingredients like grains and flour made from grains as well as any of foods on the list below, including all kinds of beans and lentils.

Common foods that are high in starch:

Beans	Fried-food	Potato chips
Bread	breading	Potatoes
Cakes	Lentils	Pretzels
Cereal	Oatmeal	Rice
Cookies	Pasta	Sweet potatoes
Crackers	Pies	

· Vegetables are classified as starchy and nonstarchy, and only certain starchy vegetables need to be avoided at night. Among the starchy vegetables, the biggest culprits are root vegetables, most notably potatoes. One large potato can contain more than 50 grams of starch, which your body will have difficulty using up in the evening. But don't forget: this doesn't mean you can't eat potatoes! You should just avoid them at dinner.

Meanwhile, certain other vegetables that are technically considered starchy contain a significantly lower amount per serving than most root vegetables. Let's call them low-starch starchy vegetables. These include butternut squash, which has only about 15 grams of starch per cup. (Acorn and pumpkin squashes have a similar amount.) These options are fine to eat in the evening as well as throughout the day.

As for the group of nonstarchy vegetables, which includes most flowering and leafy varieties? They contain little to no starch—dig in at any meal.

Starchy vegetables to avoid in the evening:

Arrowroot	Green peas	Yams
Cassava	Potatoes	
Corn	Taro	

Starchy vegetables that are okay in the evening:

Acorn squash	Lima beans	Pumpkin
Butternut squash	Parsnips	Water chestnuts

Eat all of your starches before 4 p.m.

This is a great example of how the 4 × 4 Diet doesn't necessarily eliminate foods from your diet. You want to eat starches? Not a problem—have at it, until after lunchtime. Eat that whole-wheat toast with your breakfast omelette; enjoy that sweet potato wrap for lunch. Your cutoff time should be late afternoon, around 3 or 4 p.m. As your activity level winds down, so should your starchy-carb intake.

According to the Institute of Medicine, most adults should get between 45 and 65 percent of their total daily calories from carbohydrates. For a 1,500-calorie diet, that's 675 to 975 calories—or, since carbs have 4 calories per gram, you should be consuming about 168 to 244 grams of carbohydrates per day. It is best to get most of these calories from "good" starches like vegetables and natural sugars.

Make sure they're the *right* starches.

Stick to whole grains, which give back to your body: they can reduce your risk of heart disease, are a good source of dietary fiber, and will keep you fueled for a few hours. Whole grains also break down more slowly and provide a slower release of energy, while sugar-laden white starches give you that energy spike and subsequent crash. White, or refined, grains also often lack dietary fiber and other nutrients, leaving you less satisfied.

Find nonstarchy alternatives for after lunch and dinner.

If pasta or potatoes are regular guests at your dinner table, this process may take some getting used to. Here's a positive way to look at it: you can take this opportunity to expand your palate. One of my clients discovered, in her early forties, that she loves peppers. She'd never considered them an option until we revamped her diet. She now regularly swaps out her starchy dinner side dishes—her go-to was mashed potatoes—for sautéed green, yellow, and red peppers. Try a new fruit every week as your afternoon snack. Create a whole Pinterest board for innovative cauliflower recipes. Get excited to learn what you might have been missing out on for years!

Here are some examples of healthier swaps to make throughout the day:

AFTERNOON OR EVENING SNACK

Was: Crackers; pretzels; chips; anything you might find in a vending machine

Switch to: A serving of your favorite fruit or vegetable with peanut butter, hummus, or reduced-sugar Greek yogurt dip; low-sodium string cheese; a handful of almonds; a protein shake; light cottage cheese

DINNER

Was: Anything that contains potatoes, pasta, rice, or bread

Switch to: Stir-Fry with Cauliflower Rice (see page 86); Mashed Cauliflower (see page 96); Zucchini Noodles (see page 93); summer squash; your favorite greens with a lean protein

DESSERT

Was: A slice of cake or pie; a chocolaty brownie; cookies

Switch to: A piece fruit; a dark chocolate square with almond butter; one serving of any 4 × 4 dessert (see page 101)

Two important notes on the classic popcorn snack

Always opt for air-popped over microwaveable bags, since even the options marketed as "healthier" contain salt and butter. There should be only one ingredient in popcorn: popcorn.

Despite being light and fluffy, popcorn does contain starch—it's coming from kernels of corn, a starchy vegetable. There's about 4 grams of starch per cup of popcorn, but like with most snacks, it's easy to eat more than just one cup per sitting. Those starches add up.

So keep on passing the popcorn—but make sure it's air-popped, no more than a small bowlful, and eaten in the afternoon so you can use up those starches before bedtime.

Your body uses starches as a source of energy, which is why you need them in the morning and afternoon: up until the evening hours is when you're most active. Cut off your starch intake in the late afternoon since, instead of burning them as energy, your body has a better chance of storing them as fat.

Don't mistake hunger for thirst! Before reaching for that snack or second helping, drink a glass of water and then give it up to twenty minutes to kick in.

CLEAN HABIT #2: Cut Back on Sugar

Just like starch, sugar is a carbohydrate that your body uses as energy. (Reminder: that's a good thing!) But when it's not used correctly—that is, when you consume too much of it in one sitting or gradually over time—it can lead to wacky blood sugar levels, weight gain, and heart disease, among other serious health issues. So that sweet tooth of yours? Let's extract it. This process starts with finding the right kinds and proper amount of sugar to eat.

Sugar comes in two forms: natural and added. Both are found in tons of common foods, both contribute calories to those foods, and subsequently both supply your body with energy. But that's where their similarities end.

Natural sugar is found in fruits (where it's called fructose) as well as in milk products (where it's known as lactose). The sugar itself doesn't add much in terms of vitamins or other nutrients, but it's usually surrounded by a clean and/or nutrient-rich food like a banana or a glass of milk. In other words, natural sugar is not inherently bad for you—if you're consuming it, you're by default eating something relatively healthy. So don't worry too much about limiting natural sugar; just eat it earlier in the day so you have time to use up the energy it gives you. (Warning: one of my clients ate basically only fruit for ten days and gained seven pounds. I did not approve this or even know about it! She only confessed when I asked her about it. She assumed that because she was eating fruit, it was healthy. For the record, fruit is only *part of* a well-balanced diet.)

Added sugar is the real troublemaker. It's routinely added during food prep or processing and, for most people, it makes whatever it touches taste much better. So much better that the second it hits your taste buds, it shoots a message to your brain's reward center, which releases a flood of a feel-good chemical called dopamine. Your brain is jolted into a state of bliss, all because you sank your teeth into a tasty treat. The effect is so strong that it has been compared to that of drugs and alcohol.

Also as with drugs and alcohol, the increase in dopamine levels you get when you consume sugar makes you immediately want more of whatever gave you this incredible rush—another glass of iced tea, another cupcake. **But, unlike naturally sweetened foods like fruit and milk, foods with added sugar are definitively bad because they contribute calories and little to no nutrients.** And the more foods with added sugars and empty calories you eat, the harder it is to get the nutrients you need without blowing your daily calorie budget.

The reward center of your brain is as much of a pleasure center as it is a dangerous playground. If you stimulate it too much, you can get yourself in trouble. Associating your indulgence meal as a reward for your hard work can lead to your brain getting greedy when you're not supposed to be indulging. It'll try to tell you, "I've worked hard and my reward shall be this entire carton of ice cream—I deserve it!" Leave "rewards" for the dogs; instead, see it as an evening to chill out and enjoy a couple of slices of pizza.

See where this is going? It's double trouble: eating all these processed foods means you're consuming more calories and sugar, and it also means you're more likely to *keep eating* those processed foods in order to get your sugar fix. Just as with starches, these calories can lead to an accumulation of stored body fat and weight gain if you don't burn them off. And *that* can lead to obesity, heart disease, diabetes, and even some cancers. This is what I meant about added sugar stirring up trouble.

Compounding all of this is the fact that foods with added sugar are *everywhere*. Manufacturers have capitalized on our sugar addiction and add it to all kinds of processed foods. If it comes in a box, bag, bottle, or jar, it's likely high in added sugar: Soda. Ice cream. Pasta. Energy drinks. Candy. Cereal. Sauces. In fact, an average of 16 percent of the total calories in an American's diet comes from added sugar.

So how much sugar *should* you be eating? **According to the American Heart Association, adult women should consume no more than 6 teaspoons, or about 24 grams, of sugar per day; men are allowed slightly more, 9 teaspoons, or about 36 grams.** But here's a mind-boggling stat: most Americans consume more than 22 teaspoons of added sugar per day. That's nearly four times the recommended amount for women! For context, there's about 33 grams of sugar in one 12-ounce can of Coke—that's about 8 teaspoons of sugar. If you're a woman, that's more than you should be consuming in an entire day.

Sugar is synonymous with cavities for good reason—according to a 2014 study, it's the only cause of tooth decay. Researchers from University College London and the London School of Hygiene and Tropical Medicine studied global public health records and found that people whose diet contained almost no sugar were extremely unlikely to have tooth decay—only 2 percent of the sample, taken from people in Nigeria, experienced it. Meanwhile, 92 percent of Americans have experienced tooth decay.

And because it's a carb, sugar affects your energy, also called your blood sugar level. Eating sweets will cause an immediate spike in energy followed by a crash; what you want instead is a consistent amount of energy throughout the day. The answer lies in natural sugar sources, since when you eat those, you're also getting essential nutrients. But even natural sugar should be eaten early in the day, when you need that energy and have time to burn it off. Check out the delicious 4 × 4 Breakfast Recipes on page 76.

Here's another approach: the American Heart Association also recommends consuming no more than 100 calories a day from added sugar for most women and no more than 150 calories a day for most men. To calculate the amount of calories from sugar in a product, multiply the number of grams by 4. Let's go back to the 12-ounce Coke can example: it contains 33 grams of sugar and therefore 132 calories. If you're a woman, that's one-third over your daily allowance, all from one drink.

The 4 × 4 solution: **Reduce your sugar intake at every chance, not just sporadically throughout the week**. In this book, I'll help you do just that, without making your taste buds miserable. Cutting back on the added sugars in your diet—that is, making your diet as clean as possible—frees up calories that can then be used on healthy, nutrient-dense foods. Think of it as getting more nutritional bang for your buck.

How to tell if a food is high in added sugar

When it comes to sugar, looking at the nutrition label won't help much: the number of grams listed under the sugar content includes both natural and added kinds. You want to know the specific *added* sugar content, because that's what you need to avoid. So look at the ingredients list and watch out for these words— they're code for "added sugar":

Brown sugar	Honey	Sugar molecules
Cane juice	Invert sugar	ending in "-ose"
Cane syrup	Malt sugar	(dextrose,
Corn sweetener	Malt syrup	fructose, glucose,
Corn syrup	Molasses	lactose, maltose,
Fruit juice	Raw sugar	sucrose)
concentrates	Sugar	Syrup
High-fructose corn		
syrup		

Note: ingredients are listed on the nutrition label in descending order of weight. If any of the preceding words are among the first two or three listed, that means sugar is one of the major ingredients—and that you should find another option.

Common foods that are high in sugar

Added sugar:
(Avoid these as much as possible)

Baked goods (especially store-bought)	Cereal	Pasta sauces
	Dressings	Soda
	Energy drinks	Sweets
Barbecue sauces	Fruit drinks	
Candy	Ketchup	

Natural sugar:
(Be aware of the serving size and try to eat earlier in the day)

Apples	Figs	Pineapple
Bananas	Grapes	Raisins
Cherries	Mangoes	
Dates	Milk	

How to get into the 4 × 4 habit of cutting back on added sugar

Limit your per-serving intake to 5 grams.
When you're buying processed foods, choose ones that have no more than 5 grams of added sugar per serving. If a food is processed and doesn't contain milk or fruit products, the bulk of its sugar content is likely added rather than natural. The sneakiest sugar-laden foods don't taste sweet. A half cup of Prego traditional tomato sauce, for example, contains 10 grams of sugar yet doesn't immediately jump to mind as a serious offender. If you can't let go of premade red sauce, use it as your cheat meal for a few weeks until you find a healthier substitute that you like.

Be mindful of serving sizes.
A box of cereal may say it's low in sugar, but the serving size is half a cup. Who actually eats only a half cup of cereal at a time?!

You're more likely to be filling your bowl with one to two cups of cereal, which is two to four times the serving size—and no longer low in sugar. And unless you're eating that cereal dry, you're adding at least 6 more grams of sugar (in lactose form) with a half cup of nonfat milk.

Dried fruits can be a sugar trap! Make sure you opt for dried fruit with no added sugar, and note the difference in serving size. One serving of fresh fruit is 1 cup, and one serving of dried fruit is ¼ cup. Fresh and dried often offer similar amounts of nutrients, but fresh fruit contains more water—so it'll leave you feeling fuller, longer.

Read all wording on the packaging extra carefully.

You may think you're making healthy choices at the grocery store, but food manufacturers' wording can be misleading. (That's often intentional on their part.) Straight from the American Heart Association, here's what some popular phrases actually mean:

Sugar free: It contains less than 0.5 gram of sugar per serving.

Reduced sugar or *less sugar:* It contains at least 25 percent less sugar per serving compared to a standard serving size of the traditional variety.

No added sugars or *without added sugars:* No sugars or sugar-containing ingredients, such as juice or dry fruit, have been added during processing.

Low sugar: This phrase is not defined by the American Heart Association or the U.S. Food and Drug Administration (FDA). It is not allowed as a claim on food labels.

The bottom line on sugar

It's ironic how something that tastes so sweet is actually anything but sweet for your body when you eat too much of it. Cutting back on sugar—not cutting it out completely—will produce results quickly; for some of my clients, it's been the fastest route to dropping pounds and gaining energy. Your game plan: get your sugar from natural sources like fruits and milk, and limit any processed foods you eat to those that have 5 grams of added sugar or less per serving. Breaking your sugar addiction will help combat potential health issues like weight gain and heart disease. That's a much sweeter deal.

CLEAN HABIT #3: Cut Back on Sodium

Your immediate reaction to this clean habit might be "But I don't add table salt to my meals!" And if that's the case, you're already in the right mind-set. But there's more work involved in this clean eating habit, because the salt shaker isn't where most of your sodium intake comes from. Similar to sugar, it's already in the processed food you're eating. Frustrating, right? But sodium is also easy to identify, making it easy to know what to avoid.

What you need to know about sodium and your body

As with the stars of the previous two clean eating habits, starches and sugar, you do need a bit of sodium in your diet. It plays an important role in transmitting nerve impulses and muscle contractions, it teams up with potassium to keep your body's water balance in check, and it helps control your blood pressure. For all of that to run smoothly, the U.S. Department of Agriculture (USDA) recommends in its Dietary Guidelines for Americans that most people consume no more than 2,300 milligrams of sodium per day. An important note: that recommended amount drops to 1,500 milligrams if you are fifty-one or older, if you are black, or if you have high blood pressure, diabetes, or chronic kidney disease. And these recommendations are the absolute maximum amounts you should be taking in daily. **I tell most of my clients to set their limit slightly lower than the USDA's normal recommendation: 2,000 milligrams of sodium per day.**

Sodium intake is a huge problem in the United States in particular, and it can be summed up in one astonishing stat: the average American consumes 3,400 milligrams of sodium per day—that's 1,000 milligrams more the USDA's recommendation and 1,400 milligrams more than my recommendation.

All of that excess sodium is wreaking havoc on your body, inside and out, because it makes you retain water. In the short term, it leaves you feeling bloated and looking puffy everywhere from your cheeks to your fingers to your ankles. (One of my clients describes it as "the Marshmallow Man look.") It also adds a layer of puffiness over any muscle development you are achieving through exercise, making your hard work seemingly futile. And it can mess with other parts of your body, like swelling up your joints and tightening your hamstrings.

Over time, it gets worse. The excess fluid in your system places additional strain on your heart and can subsequently increase your blood pressure, which is one of the leading causes of heart disease and stroke. According to the Centers for Disease Control and Prevention (CDC), nearly 800,000 people die each year from these diseases—that's one out of every three deaths in the United States. And more than 200,000 of these deaths could be prevented by making healthier choices, like reducing sodium intake.

Clearly, something has to change. But the answer isn't simply removing the salt shaker from the dinner table ... because the problem isn't stemming from your kitchen. Or from you, at all. The blame falls squarely on just about everyone else: according to the CDC, Americans get most of their daily sodium—more than 75 percent—from processed and restaurant foods.

When it comes to maintaining a healthy blood pressure, potassium is the yin to sodium's yang. According to the CDC, consuming enough potassium each day can help balance out the negative effects that sodium has on your blood pressure. The recommended daily amount of potassium is 4,700 milligrams, but you can't just load up on avocados or bananas and expect dazzling results the next time you measure your blood pressure— you still have to lower your sodium intake.

When it comes to processed foods, manufacturers add salt and other sodium-containing additives to make the food taste better as well as to give it a longer shelf life. And that appeal to your taste buds keeps you coming back for more the next time you stock up on groceries. Restaurants, meanwhile, serve not only huge portions of food but huge amounts of sodium in those huge portions, even in so-called healthy options like salads. (Many fast-food restaurants and diners don't make their own salad dressings. Just one tablespoon of regular premade Caesar dressing contains 156 milligrams of sodium, or 7 percent of your recommended daily amount.)

Be wary of foods that don't taste particularly salty yet are high in sodium, like grains and baked goods. One slice of white bread, for example, can contain 170 milligrams of sodium—make it a whole sandwich and you're already at 17 percent of the 2,000 milligrams of sodium you should be eating per day. And that's not counting any other ingredients between those pieces of bread!

We could all use some uplifting information right about now. So consider this: studies have demonstrated that when people are given a diet that's lower in sodium than they're used to, after a month or two, they begin to prefer the lower-sodium foods. Not only that, but when they go back and try the "old" (i.e., high-sodium) food later on, it actually tastes too salty for their liking. (It's kind of like how your eyes will adjust to the dark after a few minutes.) These findings are crucial because it means you can train your taste buds to *enjoy* healthier foods.

The 4 × 4 solution: **Reduce your sodium intake at every meal, not just sporadically throughout the week, and your taste buds will adjust accordingly.** And that's the ideal end goal: to be eating all these clean, nutritious foods because they give you pleasure— not because some expert told you to. Your target intake is no more than 2,000 milligrams of sodium per day.

How to tell if a food is high in sodium

- Check the nutrition label. Foods that are listed as having 5 percent or less sodium content per serving are considered low in sodium—these are the foods you want to fill your grocery cart with. Anything above 20 percent for sodium is considered high. As always, don't forget to calculate how many servings you're actually eating.

· In addition to the sodium listed on the nutrition label, you may see certain phrases elsewhere on the packaging. As with foods made with less sugar, there are different levels of low-sodium food. According to the FDA, they include the following:

  · *Salt free* or *sodium free:* It has less than 5 milligrams of sodium per serving.

  · *Very low sodium:* It has 35 milligrams of sodium or less per serving.

  · *Low sodium:* It has 140 milligrams of sodium or less per serving.

  · *Reduced sodium:* It has at least 25 percent less sodium than the original product.

  · *Light in sodium* or *lightly salted:* It has at least 50 percent less sodium than the regular product.

  · *No salt added* or *unsalted:* No salt was added during processing, but it is not necessarily sodium free—so check the nutrition label's sodium content.

  · *The American Heart Association Heart-Check mark:* It meets the FDA's sodium limits and supplies beneficial nutrients, making it a well-rounded choice.

· Make sure none of these words are on the package: *cured, canned, dried, instant,* or *saltwater.* These are high-sodium red flags—drop the package and run!

Common foods that are high in sodium:

Bacon	Cereal	Pickles
Bagels	Cheese	Potato chips
Baked goods	Crackers	Pretzels
Barbecue sauce	Cured meats	Queso
Blended coffee drinks	Dried beef	Salad dressing
Breads	Fish sauce	Salsa
Canned soups	Marinades	Salted nuts
Canned vegetables	Olives	Sauerkraut

| Soy sauce | Tomato sauce | Worcestershire sauce |
| Spaghetti sauce | Tortilla chips | |

How to get into the 4 × 4 habit of cutting back on sodium

Ration out your daily sodium intake.
I tell my clients to consume no more than 2,000 milligrams of sodium per day, which is less than the USDA's guidelines. A smart tactic is to break that up proportionately among your meals: about 500 milligrams at breakfast, lunch, and dinner and about 250 milligrams at each snack. All of my 4 × 4 recipes in Chapter 7 follow these guidelines.

Commit to cutting out processed foods.
The easiest way to control your sodium intake is to control the ingredients in your food. That means minimizing the amount of food you eat at restaurants and maximizing the amount of food you prepare with unprocessed ingredients at home. Turn to page 75 for a ton of recipes that my family and I—and now many of my clients and friends—make and eat regularly.

One super-helpful hint when you're stocking up on healthy ingredients: shop on the perimeter of the grocery store because that's where you'll find all the fresh stuff, like produce, seafood, and meat. (I'll bring up this point again and give you a couple other shopping tips in Chapter 6.)

It's perfectly fine to buy some processed foods, especially when you're first dipping your toes into the clean lifestyle and whenever it's time for a cheat meal. When you do, always grab the version with the lowest amount of sodium—remember that you're looking for 5 percent or less sodium content.

Experiment with herbs, seasonings, and spices.
Who said salt (or sugar) is the only way to add flavor? Now that you're making more of your own food, it's time to get creative. Raid your spice rack or the selection at your grocery store—Mrs. Dash is a brand with great zero- and low-sodium seasoning op-

tions. You can also experiment with liquids like lemon juice and low-sodium broths. See page 58 for many more ideas.

Continue to drink lots of water.
If you do end up eating an especially salty meal, drink water immediately to help flush it out of your system. As with sugar, salty foods will leave you craving even more salty foods, throwing you back into that vicious cycle. (It's no coincidence that the Pringles tagline is "Once you pop, you can't stop." The manufacturers of those salty chips not only know what they're doing—they're rubbing it in!) Remember that you're shooting to drink half your body weight in ounces of water per day.

If you're going out to eat, pick a place that makes food from scratch.
Fast-food and chain restaurants are especially likely to have high sodium levels since many of their meals are prepared ahead of time, making it impossible to adjust or remove the guilty ingredients. Find smaller local eateries that are independently owned and where the staff cooks the food to order. (For more tips on eating out, see page 54.)

The bottom line on sodium

Unless you're already actively reducing your sodium intake, you're probably consuming too much of it—and setting yourself up for bloat today and heart disease and stroke down the road. Most sodium comes from processed foods like packaged snacks, breads, and sauces, so the easiest way to remove it from your diet is to switch over to clean, naturally low-sodium foods. Since it's not realistic to expect this to happen overnight, start by reading the nutrition labels and chipping away at your sodium intake meal by meal. Your end goal should be to consume no more than 2,000 milligrams per day.

CLEAN HABIT #4: Cut Back on Alcohol

If you abstain from drinking, for whatever reason, congrats—you've already nailed the final clean eating habit. If you do indulge in a drink from time to time (or even more frequently), limiting your intake is the final piece of the clean eating puzzle. When it's abused, alcohol does a lot of damage to your body while providing it with exactly zero nutrients. These reasons and more are why it shouldn't be a large part of your diet.

What you need to know about alcohol and your body

No surprise here: heavy alcohol consumption can take a *serious* toll on your body. Let's start by exploring how it affects your major organs and important bodily functions:

- The first thing many people think of is the liver, and rightly so—heavy drinking can lead to a fatty or inflamed liver, alcoholic hepatitis, scarring, fibrosis, and cirrhosis. It's also a primary cause of liver cancer.
- Alcohol can damage your heart, too, causing issues such as cardiomyopathy, irregular heartbeat, stroke, and high blood pressure.
- Then there are alcohol's effects on your brain and its communication pathways. In the short term, it's responsible for memory lapse, blurred vision, slurred speech, and hindered balance and mobility—better known as being sloppy drunk. Years of heavy drinking can cause more permanent cognitive damage, either directly or indirectly thanks to vitamin deficiencies.
- Pancreatitis and pancreatic cancer are other diseases linked to heavy drinking.
- Finally, your immune system weakens with excessive drinking, meaning you're more likely to contract infections and diseases like pneumonia and tuberculosis.

I don't want to minimize these issues, at all. They're serious conditions, they can ultimately be deadly, and you should be informed of the damage that alcohol is capable of doing. But **my reason for cutting back on alcohol is much simpler: It's full of empty calories and can make you gain weight.** In a way, alcohol is the worst kind of offender, because unlike starches, sugar, and sodium, your body doesn't need it to function. You're consuming truly empty calories with every sip—it's like liquid candy. Not convinced yet? In the following chart listing the amount of calories and sugar in different kinds of alcohol, picture one last column across the top called NUTRIENTS. Underneath it, for every type of alcohol, you could fill in a zero.

According to the CDC, the term "heavy drinking" is defined as consuming 15 drinks or more per week for men and 8 drinks or more per week for women.

Type of Alcohol	Serving Size	Number of Calories	Grams of Sugar
Champagne/ sparkling wine	14-ounce glass	80–90	Varies; stick to dry options
Gin	1 ounce	64	0
Red wine	15-ounce glass	125–200	Varies; stick to dry options
Regular beer	1 can or bottle	153–170	0
Rum (80 proof)	1 ounce	64	0
Scotch	1 ounce	64	0
Tequila (80 proof)	1 ounce	64	0
Vodka	1 ounce	64	0
Whiskey/bourbon (80 proof)	1 ounce	64	0
White wine	15-ounce glass	110–170	Varies; stick to dry options

These values are estimated because nutrition information is not required to be listed on alcohol.

The more you drink, the more calories and sugar you consume. And, simply put, these actions fuel your sugar addiction. Making it worse is that alcohol lowers your judgment, inhibitions, and willpower—that goes back to its effect on your brain—making you far more likely to accompany those drinks with unhealthy food, like pizza topped with pools of grease. And it continues the next morning when you decide that the only cure for your hangover is an oversize high-sodium breakfast. What a mess!

The 4 × 4 solution: **Have two to three drinks per week, maximum.** Yes, it may be a drastic reduction if you're used to drinking in social situations or if you work in an industry where you're surrounded by open bars. (Also: wedding season.) This step is the hardest one for some of my clients, and it may be for you, too. The tools and tactics below will help get you there.

How to get into the 4 × 4 habit of cutting back on alcohol

Resolve not to drink on a whim.

At the beginning of each week, assess your personal and professional obligations and note which ones could potentially involve alcohol: a dinner date, a work function, a weekend birthday bash. Which parties or events will you designate as your chance to (smartly) indulge in that three-drink max? Choose wisely, and stand by your decision.

Treat your taste buds.

Speaking of indulging, you should be drinking because you enjoy the actual taste of the alcohol—not because it takes the edge off or because you feel like you need it to talk to a blind date. Reducing your intake will allow you to enjoy it even more, since it's now a treat instead of the norm. Sip that occasional glass of wine or martini slowly, and really savor it.

WHEN YOU'RE NOT DRINKING:

Recruit a nondrinking buddy. Or a whole group of nondrinking buddies. If you surround yourself with people you can have fun with in any situation, you'll be less tempted to order an alcoholic beverage. In the best-case scenario, you'll inspire your friends and family to cut back on their alcohol intake, too.

Make it so that you *can't* drink. Meet up with friends at places that don't even serve alcohol, like a park, coffee shop, or bowling alley. Don't keep booze in your house. And volunteer to be the designated driver for the evening, if that's an option. Sometimes all it takes is just informing one person that you're planning on not imbibing—you'll have someone else holding you accountable.

Find tasty nonalcoholic alternatives. When alcohol is involved in a celebratory occasion, like a holiday party or engagement brunch, you can still toast with a special drink. Here's another chance to get creative with ingredients: make your own mocktails with your favorite zero- or low-calorie sparkling water, fruits, and herbs.

Mocktails

Mix one of these liquids:

Club soda/ soda water	Green tea Mineral water	Seltzer water

With one or more of these fruits/vegetables:

Acai	Honeydew	Pear
Blood orange	Kiwi	Persimmon
Blueberries	Lemon	Pineapple
Cantaloupe	Lime	Pomegranate
Cherries	Lychee	Raspberries
Coconut	Mango	Strawberries
Cucumber	Oranges	Watermelon
Grapefruit		

And/or these herbs:

Basil	Ginger	Mint
Cilantro	Honey	Rosemary
Elderflower	Lavender	

And/or these sweeteners:

Agave nectar	Stevia	Truvia

Diet soda

Diet tonic water

Energy drinks (like Red Bull)

Liquids with the word "cocktail" on the package

Premade mixers (like margarita, piña colada, mudslide, or Bloody Mary mixes)

Simple syrup

Soda

Sour mix

Sweetened fruit juices (like cranberry juice); a splash is okay

Tomato juice

Tonic water

Sample Mocktail

1 cup club soda
A squeeze of lemon
A squeeze of lime
A splash of agave nectar or orange juice

WHEN YOU DO DRINK:

Make smart, healthy choices. Opt for these low-calorie/low-sugar cocktails:

- Vodka soda with a splash of cranberry and a lime
- Tequila on the rocks with a lime
- Light beer (unless there's one *really* good regular beer that you love)
- White wine
- Any of your mocktails with one shot of vodka

Sample Cocktail

1 shot vodka
1 cup club soda (optional)
A squeeze of lemon
A squeeze of lime
A splash of agave nectar or orange juice

You can get creative here, too, as long as you stick with healthy ingredients and, in general, lighter-colored liquids.

Alternate with water. If you're having more than one of your allotted two to three drinks on the same night—or if you're counting a few drinks as one of your weekly indulgences—this one's for you. Alternating each drink with water will serve three important functions: it'll slow down your alcohol intake, it'll hydrate you, and it has the potential to prevent a nasty hangover the next morning.

The bottom line on alcohol

If you don't drink, you're one step ahead of the game. If you do drink regularly, you need to start seeing alcohol as a treat that's meant to be indulged in only a couple of times a week, tops. In addition to all the other damage booze does to your body, consider the sugar and calories it contains—would you have five back-to-back desserts without batting an eye? The only difference with booze is that it contains even fewer nutrients than a slice of cake.

FOOD ON THE GO

Your home, especially your kitchen, is a controlled environment. There's nothing in your fridge, freezer, or pantry that you didn't put there. But once you walk out your front door? All bets are off. Temptation in the form of unhealthy foods is everywhere: salty potato chips in vending machines, sugar-loaded candy in the checkout line, glazed donuts in the break room at work. And the size of the portions at most restaurants? Those are not only uncontrollable—they're out of control.

Unfortunately, you can't prevent this stuff from popping into your everyday life. Here's what you *can* do: be prepared so that you're not tempted to succumb to their magnetic pull. That means taking a few minutes ahead of time—in the morning before you leave your house or the night before you leave for a trip—and stocking your bag, purse, carry-on, whatever. When you're armed with healthy options that you look forward to eating, you have no excuse to give in to the health hazards of the outside world.

On-the-Go Snacks

An apple

A banana with a squeeze pack of almond butter

Your favorite sliced vegetables (such as peppers, celery, carrots, and mushrooms) with a small container of hummus

A small plastic bowl of light air-popped popcorn

Frozen grapes

A piece of light string cheese

Brown rice cakes with a smear of peanut or almond butter or a drizzle of honey

Protein powder in a shaker—don't mix it with water until you're
ready to drink it

A snack bar with 5 grams of added sugar or less

A Whole-Wheat Banana Wrap or Apple Wrap (see page 100)

A Banana Blueberry Muffin (see page 99)

A handful of Oil-Free Sautéed Almonds (see page 98) or Oven-
Roasted Spicy Almonds (see page 99)

Homemade trail mix with your favorite unsalted nuts and dried
berries (one idea: raw almonds, reduced-sugar cranberries,
and whole-wheat Chex cereal)

A small plastic container of berries (so they don't get smashed)

Old-fashioned oats with fried egg whites and strawberries

On-the-Go Lunches

Avocado whole-wheat pita or turkey pita with tomatoes, sprouts,
and hummus

Yup, oatmeal again—it's my favorite breakfast *and* lunch! If you're
grabbing it from a café or kiosk, be aware of the sugar content
and type.

Natural peanut butter and a drizzle of honey on whole-grain
bread

Quinoa tabouli in a plastic container

EATING HEALTHY AT RESTAURANTS

Eat before you go. Nibble on some almonds, an apple, or a small salad to keep yourself from overeating when you finally sit down for your meal.

Drink water before and during your meal. Make sure you're not mistaking hunger for dehydration. (For other signs of dehydration, flip back to page 9.)

Cut the cheese. Order dishes without it or with a much smaller amount.

Limit your alcohol consumption. Nurse your drink so you don't overindulge, and drink a full glass of water between alcoholic beverages. This helps you slow down on your booze intake, plus you'll rehydrate your body. Alcohol can weaken your willpower and turn a restaurant menu into a feeding frenzy. More on these dangers—and why cutting back on alcohol is the final 4 × 4 habit—on page 46.

Beware of dressings and toppings. Just because it's called a salad doesn't mean healthy. Dressings—especially creamy ones like ranch and Caesar—are loaded with sodium, fat, and sugar, so order the lightest option available on the side and use it in moderation. As for the toppings, stay away from notorious calorie and fat bombs, such as cheese, croutons, and bacon.

Choose veggies wisely. Grilled, roasted, and steamed vegetables are a yes. Sautéed is a maybe, depending on the kind of oil being used. Fried vegetables are a firm nope.

Avoid butter and oil whenever possible. Order fish, chicken, and veggies sans any kind of oil. At Mexican restaurants, I order fajitas without the sizzle.

Watch portion size. A few tactics: Order an appetizer as your meal with a side of veggies. Or order an entrée and divide it in half the second it's in front of you, then share it or eat it the next day for lunch. Want an appetizer? Look at the salads and sides, which are often healthier than the official appetizer offerings.

Enlist your server. Request that the bread basket or chips on the table be removed after everyone has had one serving. Better yet, have it whisked away before you even sit down.

Learn the lingo. Watch for words like *alfredo, breaded, crispy, dipped, loaded, panfried, panko, smothered,* and *tempura*—these are menu-speak for "lots of fat, calories, and sodium."

CHAPTER 5

All-Star Ingredients and Kitchen Tools

As much as I love experimenting in my kitchen and trying to come up with clean (and yummy) variations on my family's favorite meals, there are several ingredients that I find myself using over and over again. They're comfort foods in the sense that I know I can count on them to be as nutritious as they are versatile. It's a similar deal with kitchen appliances—while I can admire shiny new gadgets and fancy upgraded models, I have an arsenal of small, no-nonsense tools that I rely on for all sorts of cooking situations. Here are my kitchen essentials—and how they can help you embrace a clean lifestyle.

All-Star Ingredients

A lot of people ask what's in my pantry, and my answer is simple, healthy foods—lots of them. Below are ten ingredients that I keep stocked in my kitchen because of their versatility and wide-ranging health benefits. Going through the checkout with nine dozen eggs, two huge packs of sliced raw almonds, and enough chicken to feed a high school football team may seem absurd, but these are the staples that keep my active family of four eating clean and feeling good.

All-Star Ingredient #1: Unsweetened Almond Milk

Almond milk has long been a go-to for people who are vegan, are lactose intolerant, or simply don't like the taste of dairy products. I don't fall into any of those categories—I use almond milk for its all-around nutritional awesomeness. For starters, it contains no cholesterol, saturated fat, or added sugar. One cup of certain brands also supplies about 50 percent of your recommended daily amount of vitamin E, which protects your body from damaging free radicals. Unsweetened almond milk has only about 30 calories per cup, compared to about 86 in skim milk, 122 in 2 percent milk, and a whopping 146 in whole milk. (Calories don't always tell the whole story, but that sure is an impressive stat.)

One thing to keep in mind is that almond milk is nowhere near as protein-rich as cow's milk—it has just 1 gram, compared to 8 grams in cow's milk—despite being made from almonds. (The protein gets strained out in the conversion from nut to milk.) But as a whole, almond milk is packed with more nutrients than cow's milk and offers a nutty taste and silky texture that makes it feel indulgent. So if you haven't tried it yet, it's worth a taste test.

4 × 4 recipes that use unsweetened almond milk:
- Whole-Wheat Crepes (see page 76)
- Apple Cinnamon Oatmeal Pecan Crunch (see page 77)
- Veggie, Egg, and Quinoa Casserole (see page 79)
- Lemon Pancakes with Blueberry Compote (see page 80)
- Mashed Cauliflower (see page 96)
- Cookie Dough Hummus (see page 102)

Other ways to use unsweetened almond milk:
- Over cereal
- In baked goods
- In any smoothie

- In mashed potatoes
- In French toast batter
- In coffee

All-Star Ingredient #2: Kale

I could talk about kale forever. I could also eat kale forever. And I do, sort of—I work it into my diet on a near-daily basis. Kale is commonly referred to as a superfood, and it certainly lives up to the hype: it is bursting with nutrients, like vitamin A, vitamin C, and calcium. (One cup contains twice the recommended daily amount of vitamin A and well over the recommended daily amount of vitamin C—it's a bit of an overachiever.) Raw kale also has tons of dietary fiber—about 1.3 grams per cup—which is key for making you feel full, keeping your blood sugar in check, and normalizing your bowel movements. It's high in protein, too, containing about 2 grams per cup; you'll also get a solid dose of folate, which plays a role in brain development, and iron, which is crucial in supplying your body with oxygen. For these reasons and more, kale is not only worthy of its superfood status—it's approaching superhero territory. (Like most superheroes, kale has a tragic flaw. Raw, whole kale is very tough, so it's best eaten after being chopped, pulsed, or sautéed.)

4 × 4 recipes that use kale:
- Kale Quinoa Asian Salad (see page 83)
- Asian Tuna Steak on a Bed of Sautéed Kale (see page 91)
- Kale Salad with Chicken (see page 94)
- Sweet Green Smoothie (see page 105) or any other smoothie

Other ways to use kale:
- Pulsed in a food processor as the base of any salad
- Processed or sautéed with garlic salt
- As kale chips
- On top of pizza

All-Star Ingredient #3: Salt-Free Seasonings and Herbs

Remember when I told you that many of my clients say they don't eat healthy foods because they don't taste good? That excuse ends with your spice rack, which can add limitless flavor combinations to any dish.

One of the most surprisingly effective offerings I've found is the taco seasoning from a brand called Mrs. Dash. This product is a gem because it's one of the few store-bought taco seasonings that contains no salt. It adds a little kick to ground beef and ground turkey, whether you're using that meat for tacos or not. And a little goes a long way—I usually use only about one-half or one-third of a packet for each recipe.

My go-to seasonings and spices:

Cayenne pepper	Garlic powder	Rosemary
Chili powder	Onion powder	Salt-free taco
Cilantro	Oregano	seasoning
Dill	Red pepper flakes	

4 × 4 recipes that use salt-free taco seasoning:
- Salt-free taco seasoning in Stuffed Quinoa Peppers (see page 85) and Lettuce Wrap Tacos (see page 95)
- Cumin and paprika in Roasted Vegetable Hash (see page 76)
- Red pepper flakes in Sautéed Spinach and Scrambled Egg Burrito for Two (see page 80)
- Cilantro in Rice Paper Wraps (see page 83), Stuffed Quinoa Peppers (see page 85), and Quinoa Tabouli Salad (see page 86)
- Basil in Spicy Bahn Mi Wrap (see page 84)
- Cayenne pepper in Sautéed Brussels Sprouts (see page 89)
- Lemon pepper in Lemon Pepper Cod (see page 93)

Other ways to use seasonings:
- Salt-free taco seasoning in Mexican lasagna or fish tacos
- Cilantro and garlic on shrimp

- Red pepper flakes on zucchini noodles
- Rosemary on roasted veggies

All-Star Ingredient #4: PB2

A powdered peanut butter substitute may not sound super appetizing, so maybe PB2's nutritional info will convince you of its all-star-worthiness: two tablespoons has 45 calories, 1.5 grams of fat, and 1 gram of sugar. That same amount of a natural creamy peanut butter spread like Jif contains 190 calories, 16 grams of fat, and 3 grams of sugar. What's not to love about all that healthiness? You don't have to use PB2 in every recipe that calls for peanut butter—you mix it with water, so it doesn't have quite the same consistency—but, as with almond milk, give this alternative a shot if you haven't yet.

4 × 4 recipes that use PB2:
- Easy Yogurt Parfait (see page 78)
- Brown rice cakes with PB2
- Peanut Butter Chocolate Protein Brownies (see page 102)
- Client Classic Smoothie (see page 105)

Other ways to use PB2:
- In any smoothie
- In yogurt
- In oatmeal
- In cookies
- In pancakes

All-Star Ingredient #5: Avocados

Where to begin with a flavorful, fleshy fruit that has been dubbed "the perfect food"? Avocados are loaded with good fats—specifically, monosaturated fats—which your body uses to lower cholesterol and absorb nutrients like vitamins A and D. They're higher in potassium than bananas, with more than 25 percent of the recommended daily amount and serious debloating capabilities. (A medium-size banana has about half that amount. Why it is still the go-to example of high-potassium foods is beyond me, but I digress.) Because of their richness and creaminess, you can sneak avocados into all sorts of recipes; they're so versatile that you can even use them as a butter substitute—see page 114 for details on that.

4 × 4 recipes that use avocados:
- Avocado Toast with Fried Egg (see page 78)
- Sautéed Spinach and Scrambled Egg Burrito for Two (see page 80)
- Root Vegetable Tacos (see page 81)
- Hummus Sandwich (see page 82)
- Rice Paper Wraps (see page 83)
- Thai Salad (see page 89)
- Lettuce Wrap Tacos (see page 95)
- Berry Creme Smoothie (see page 104)

Other ways to use avocados:
- In guacamole with pineapple, mango, or cantaloupe
- As a baking substitution for butter or oil
- As a creamy pasta sauce

All-Star Ingredient #6: Oatmeal

Oatmeal is usually chalked up as a basic breakfast food, but it deserves more credit than that. One cup, cooked, contains about 4 grams of fiber, which arms you with energy; unlike most sugary breakfast cereals, it'll keep you full for a few hours. Over time, fiber-rich foods like oatmeal can even lower your cholesterol.

And, yeah, plain oatmeal isn't the most exciting food to taste or look at—it's a trade-off for being very low in sugar and sodium. But you can use its blandness to your advantage by changing its flavor completely with a couple of other clean ingredients. Sweeten up your oatmeal by topping it with your favorite berries, or give it a savory spin by adding turkey bacon and a fried egg.

That versatility makes it easier to eat several times per week—or, in my world, several times per day. It's surprisingly portable and doesn't even need to be heated up. If you're not going to eat it for a few hours, just add a little extra water so it doesn't dry up.

Finally, make sure you're eating the healthiest variety of oatmeal: either old-fashioned oats—also called rolled oats—or steelcut oats. (The latter is less processed but takes longer to prepare.) Stay away from instant oatmeal, especially the individual packets, which usually contain an alarming amount of added sugar, salt, and other additives.

4 × 4 recipes that use oatmeal:
  · Breakfast of Champions (see page 77)
  · Apple Cinnamon Oatmeal Pecan Crunch (see page 77)
  · Tour de Breakfast (see page 79)
  · Cookie Dough Hummus (see page 102)

Other ways to use oatmeal:
  · Topped with a fried egg
  · Mixed with spices like cinnamon, cardamom, and ginger
  · Topped with nuts like walnuts, cashews, or pecans

All-Star Ingredient #7: Eggs

Like oatmeal, eggs are a versatile food that you can eat at any time of day—not just at breakfast. You may have heard mixed reviews of eggs, especially when it comes to their cholesterol content: one whole medium egg contains 186 milligrams of cholesterol, which is half of the daily recommended amount. Recent studies have been showing that eggs may not be as bad for you (and your heart) as they've been made out to be, but I play it safe by eating mostly egg whites. (All of an egg's cholesterol is found in the yolk.) You'll notice that most 4 × 4 recipes call for a combination of whole eggs and egg whites. Not only are egg whites more nutrient-dense than whole eggs, but they take on the taste of whatever food you add them to.

To separate an egg white, the only thing you'll need is a bowl. Swiftly crack the egg and allow the yolk to settle into half of the shell while the white drips into the bowl. Then transfer the yolk back and forth between the shell halves, with the goal of separating as much remaining egg white as possible. With lots of practice at the kitchen counter, even my kids have become pros.

One whole egg:	One egg white:
78 calories	17 calories
6 grams of protein	3.6 grams of protein
6 grams of fat	<0.1 gram of fat
187 grams of cholesterol	0 grams of cholesterol

4 × 4 recipes that use eggs:
- Whole-Wheat Crepes (see page 76)
- Breakfast of Champions (see page 77)
- Avocado Toast with Fried Egg (see page 78)
- Veggie, Egg, and Quinoa Casserole (see page 79)
- Tour de Breakfast (see page 79)
- Sautéed Spinach and Scrambled Egg Burrito for Two (see page 80)
- Lemon Pancakes with Blueberry Compote (see page 80)
- Chicken Tenders (see pages 87 and 88)
- Sautéed Brussels Sprouts with Fried Egg (see page 89)
- Oven-Roasted Spicy Almonds (see page 99)
- Peanut Butter Chocolate Protein Brownies (see page 102)

Other ways to use eggs:
- A batch of egg muffins
- Mixed with oatmeal
- On cinnamon toast

All-Star Ingredient #8: Almonds

Barring a tree nut allergy, almonds are the ideal snack. A handful (about twenty-three whole almonds) has about 3.5 grams of fiber and nearly 6 grams of protein, which will fill you up between meals. I usually keep a stash of baked or sautéed almonds in my house for anyone in the family to grab before heading out the door. Leaving a container of raw almonds in your car will prevent you from hitting up a fast-food drive-through in a moment of weakness. And making your own almond flour—read more about its versatility on page 109—is as easy as pressing a button on your food processor.

4 × 4 recipes that use almonds:
- Lemon Pancakes with Blueberry Compote (see page 80)
- Chicken Tenders (Traditional Flavor) (see page 87)
- Chicken Tenders (Italian Blend) (see page 88)
- Sautéed Brussels Sprouts with Fried Egg (see page 89)
- Kale Salad with Chicken (see page 94)
- Oil-Free Sautéed Almonds (see page 98)
- Oven-Roasted Spicy Almonds (see page 99)
- Peanut Butter Chocolate Protein Brownies (see page 102)
- No-Bake Individual Cheesecakes (see page 103)

Other ways to use almonds:
- In any baked good that calls for flour
- As a coating on fish like cod or halibut
- In any salad
- In a homemade batch of almond butter
- For some quick protein in oatmeal

All-Star Ingredient #9: Boneless, Skinless Chicken

Chicken is another blank-slate kind of food—you can make it taste like whatever you want it to. Start by prepping it in a healthy way—by grilling, boiling, broiling, or throwing it in a slow cooker. Then use it to add protein to any wrap, salad, sandwich, casserole, omelet, or taco you see fit. (And don't forget that it can stand on its own just fine.) When prepped ahead of time, it'll last three or four days in the fridge—other proteins, like salmon, won't last that long.

Nutritionally, one whole chicken breast yields about 34 grams of protein and only 128 milligrams of sodium. (Just make sure you're removing the fatty skin.) Chicken is on the high side when it comes to cholesterol—about 146 milligrams in one breast, which is nearly half of the daily recommended value. If you have high cholesterol, take note; if not, then savor this poultry's nutritional benefits.

4 × 4 recipes that use boneless, skinless chicken:
- Apple Cider Salad (see page 82)
- Rice Paper Wraps (see page 83)
- Spicy Bahn Mi Wrap (see page 84)
- Chicken Salad (see page 85)
- Stir-Fry with Cauliflower Rice (see page 86)
- Chicken Tenders (see pages 87 and 88)
- Chicken Caprese (see page 94)
- Kale Salad with Chicken (see page 94)

Other ways to use boneless, skinless chicken:
- In a slow cooker with low-sodium seasoning
- In any wrap, salad, sandwich, or casserole

All-Star Ingredient #10: Fresh Berries

Blueberries, blackberries, strawberries, raspberries, and cranberries may have different tastes, but they all are crammed with fiber. In one cup, strawberries have 3 grams, blueberries have 4 grams, cranberries have 5 grams, and blackberries and raspberries have a whopping 8 grams. Across the board, berries are also a stellar source of vitamin C and manganese while being low in calories. (In general, the darker the color, the better the berry.)

One nutritional component to be aware of is the amount of sugar, which varies from berry to berry—cranberries are among the lowest, with only 4 grams per cup, but blueberries contain 15 grams of sugar per cup. Luckily, since it's natural sugar rather than added sugar, you're still reaping tons of nutritional benefits.

As for berries' versatility, you can use them to sweeten whatever your stomach desires: pancakes, oatmeal, muffins, cereal, smoothies, yogurt, and more. Use them whole, purée them, mash them into a spread—or freeze them for a refreshing treat on a hot day.

4 × 4 recipes that use berries:
- Whole-Wheat Crepes (see page 76)
- Breakfast of Champions (see page 77)
- Easy Yogurt Parfait (see page 78)
- Tour de Breakfast (see page 79)
- Lemon Pancakes with Blueberry Compote (see page 80)
- Banana Blueberry Muffins (see page 99)
- Not-So-Boring Brown Rice Cake (see page 100)
- Almond Butter No-Bake Bar with Berries (see page 101)
- Berry Creme Smoothie (see page 104)
- Cocktails and mocktails (see page 50)

Other ways to use berries:
- Homemade freezer pops
- In yogurt
- In salads

All-Star Kitchen Tools

I approach kitchen equipment and workout equipment the same way: I rely on a few key versatile pieces that I am constantly finding new uses for. When I'm exercising, that equipment comes in the form of dumbbells and resistance bands; when I'm making food, the equipment comes in the form of common small to medium-size appliances. No bells and whistles, no intricately worded instruction manuals—in fact, you probably already have a couple of these tools in your own kitchen. These are five of my favorites and how to maximize their capabilities.

All-Star Tool #1: Spiralizer

This handy tool turns firm fruits and vegetables into long, noodlelike strands. The resulting dishes are hands down my favorite substitute for starchy pastas—especially for dinner meals, when you're avoiding starches.

The recipe possibilities are endless. Nearly any healthy sauce or topping you normally put on pasta will work with zucchini and squash noodles, but without all the carbs. Plus, it's quicker than making pasta since you don't have to boil water. Just spiralize a whole raw zucchini, warm up those noodles, and then top them as you would spaghetti (with olive oil, other veggies, herbs like lemon and thyme, chicken, tofu, shrimp, or grilled fish). There are high-end spiralizers from stores like Williams-Sonoma and versions that have their own infomercial. Find one that fits your budget.

4 × 4 recipes that use a spiralizer:
· Zucchini Noodles with Pesto and Tilapia (see page 93)
This is the only official 4 × 4 recipe that calls for a spiralizer, but get creative with healthy sauces to top your zucchini noodles!

Other foods on which to use a spiralizer:
· Squash
· Carrots
· Cucumbers
· Potatoes
· Apples

All-Star Tool #2: Contact Grill

Electric countertop grills can remove more than 40 percent of the fat in your meats while retaining their taste. I also rely on this tool for its ease of use—I can whip up burgers, chicken, fish, and grilled veggies in just a few minutes. And that's important when you have two hungry boys and a hungry grown man waiting for their food. A few good brands out there include George Foreman,

Cuisinart, and Breville. (Like with the all appliances, choose one that fits both your budget and countertop.)

4 × 4 recipes that use a contact grill:
- Lemon Pepper Cod (see page 93)
- Asian Tuna Steak on a Bed of Sautéed Kale (see page 91)

Other ways to use a contact grill:
- Grilling chicken
- Grilling beef
- Grilling fish, such as tuna, tilapia, and salmon

All-Star Tool #3: Food Processor

Handiest of all of today's kitchen technology is one of the most classic: the food processor. I have both a small and large food processor and can't picture my life, or meals, without either of them. They do it all—chop, shred, mix, slice, julienne, purée, and more—and they do it in seconds.

4 × 4 recipes that use a food processor:
- Stir-Fry with Cauliflower Rice (see page 86)
- Thai Salad (see page 89)
- Zucchini Noodles with Pesto and Tilapia (see page 93)
- Kale Salad with Chicken (see page 94)
- Mashed Cauliflower (see page 96)
- Cookie Dough Hummus (see page 102)
- Two-Layer Peanut Butter Brownies (see page 103)

Other ways to use a food processor:
- To blend smoothies
- To make dressings
- To make almond flour
- To make hummus

All-Star Tool #4: Quality Food Storage Containers

You probably already have a random assortment of plastic containers stashed in your kitchen cabinets—but, upon closer inspection, maybe several lids have gone missing or some of your options are actually repurposed yogurt containers. I can't stress the power of high-quality storage for your leftovers, premade foods, and meals on the go. Proper storage will help preserve the food's nutritional value and taste, so invest in a dishwasher-safe set with these key qualities:

1. Snapping lids to lock in the food and provide airtight and water-tight safekeeping

2. Color-coordinated lids to keep the different sizes organized (especially handy when you're reaching for one in a hurry)

3. Glass is the more ecofriendly version but is generally more expensive than plastic, so go with whatever fits your budget.

4 × 4 recipes that use storage containers:
- Pepper mix (see page 73)
- De-vined grapes (see page 73)
- Mixed berries (see page 73)
- Chopped romaine (see page 73)
- Leftover dressing

Other ways to use storage containers:
- All of your leftovers
- Almond flour
- Chopped nuts
- Meals on the go, like oatmeal

All-Star Tool #5: Slow Cooker

You already know that the slow cooker is one of the easiest kitchen appliances to use—often the most effort required is tossing a bunch of ingredients in the pot and going about your day. But all these years, your slow cooker has been keeping a huge secret from you: it can make so much more than the stews, pot roasts, and chili you rely on it for. We're talking everything from oatmeal to salmon to pork tenderloin to rice pudding, all in large batches that you can eat throughout the week. That kind of versatility may even make up for all the counter space it takes up.

4 × 4 recipes that use a slow cooker:
- Apple Cinnamon Oatmeal Pecan Crunch (see page 77)

Other ways to use a slow cooker:
- Any other kind of oatmeal
- Boneless chicken with a low or no-sodium marinade or low-sodium chicken broth
- Granola
- Eggplant lasagna
- Quinoa
- Sweet potatoes

CHAPTER 6

Prep Day

My family is always, always on the go. My husband and I are usually running to client sessions—he's a personal trainer as well—and our two sons bounce around from school to soccer practice to their friends' houses. That doesn't leave a lot of time for any of us to prepare meals. So I developed a system called Prep Day. It's exactly what it sounds like: once a week, we set aside a few hours to go grocery shopping and then come home and prepare as much of that food as possible for the week ahead. (For my family, Prep Day usually falls on a Monday—but pick the day that works best for your particular schedule.)

On Prep Day, there's a flurry of action going on in the kitchen: washing, slicing, mixing, chopping, baking, and roasting. It requires some ahead-of-time meal planning, since you'll need to map out a general idea of what you'll be eating (and not eating) over the next seven days, but it'll save you time later on and leave you less likely to impulse-eat a less-healthy option. In addition, it'll allow you to have at least a few moments of downtime later in the day or week when you're not worrying about healthy eating and you can finally relax. Prepping is the key to having it all.

PART 1: Grocery Shopping

Buying groceries can often be an overwhelming, stressful, and time-consuming weekly experience—but it doesn't have to be if you're well prepared. Arm yourself with a written-out shopping list plus these tips.

TIP: Always go to the same store.

When you find a grocery store that you really like, whether it's due to its proximity to your house, the frequent sales, or even the extra-friendly cashiers, make a point to become a valued, card-carrying customer. This way, you'll learn where all of your regular necessities are stocked and you won't have to go scouring the aisles for the raw nuts or the Greek yogurt. (I've actually had clients call me from the local grocery store asking where certain items are—I know the layout *that* well.) You'll be in control of the situation the second you walk inside. And, short of a major renovation, it'll stay that way.

TIP: Shop on the perimeter of the store.

It's convenient, but not a coincidence, that the healthiest foods are stocked on the perimeter of the grocery store. That's where you'll find most of the produce, meats, and dairy—essentially, all the unprocessed stuff that forms the foundation of a clean diet. You'll still need to venture into the inner aisles for items like nuts, oatmeal, and baking ingredients, but most of your time should be spent on the outskirts of the store.

TIP: Never, ever shop on an empty stomach.

You may have heard this trick before and taken it with a grain of salt. But now there's scientific evidence to back it up: Researchers gathered a group of study participants and fed half of them a snack before unleashing them in a simulated grocery store; those who shopped while hungry opted for more high-calorie items. Then the researchers followed around actual shoppers in a grocery store at a time when they were most likely to be hungry (between lunch and dinner, from 4 to 7 p.m.). They, too, chose more foods that were higher in calories. Their conclusion, in unscientific terms, is that everything looks *delicious* when you're hungry—especially processed, quick bites. So don't even put yourself in that situation. Do your grocery shopping after a meal, or grab one of the on-the-go snacks on page 52 before going to the store.

So, that's the scientific evidence. Here's my anecdotal evidence: I once made the mistake of going to the grocery store starving and ended up with a full cart in a backed-up checkout line. I became hungry-angry—hangry. If I'd had to wait just one minute longer, I easily would've abandoned my cart and walked out of the store so I could go eat. Looking back, I realized, if you're in a similar rushed, irritated state, are you going to have the mental clarity to buy the right foods? Probably not. And even if you do, will you want to prep it all the minute you get home? *Definitely* not. So schedule your grocery shopping for after a meal—and keep some healthy snacks in your glove compartment, just in case.

PART 2: The Prep

Once you've loaded up on your groceries, take them home and immediately unpack everything you plan to prep—but don't put them away. In fact, the very next thing you should do is preheat your oven, so that you're forced to keep the momentum going instead of getting sucked into your couch or other chores. The point is to do everything you can in this moment so you don't have to do it during the week, when you're really crunched for time. (In a way, you're looking out for your safety, too—chopping or sautéing while you're in a hurry is dangerous!) Since you'll have the food all ready to go in the days to come, you'll also be less tempted to eat out at a restaurant.

To Prep or Not to Prep?

My family has been practicing Prep Day for years, so by now we've gotten it down to a science. Certain foods, I've learned, are worth the time and energy you put into prepping them for the week.

Other foods *aren't* worth it—the extra money you may pay makes up for the convenience of having them pre-sliced, pre-cut, or pre-cooked. Prep Day in my household involves tackling these foods:

- **Grapes.** De-vine these delicious fruits so they're easy to access and pop in your mouth. I started doing this after seeing clients stock up on bunches and then let them sit in the fridge untouched, until they shriveled up. Never waste grapes again!
- **Peppers.** Chop up your stash of raw peppers and toss them into a container—I call this my pepper mix (creative, right?) and find myself reaching for it often. I toss it into omelettes, egg wraps, tacos, and salads. I also slice them up for easy snacking.
- **Nuts.** Bake your almonds, pecans, walnuts, pine nuts right in a row, using the 4 × 4 recipe on page 98. Keep these guys on hand for salad toppings, veggie dish toppings, and grab-and-go snacking.
- **Chicken.** Cook at least part of your weekly supply of chicken, whether your preferred method is grilling, baking, or roasting. I'm also not afraid of buying a rotisserie chicken at the grocery store and tearing off pieces sans skin throughout the week for salads, wraps, and stir-fries.
- **Romaine lettuce.** Chop up your romaine for the week's salads. I've found that buying these greens whole is slightly cheaper than buying them bagged and pre-chopped.
- **Berries.** After washing your berries, toss 'em into a clear airtight container. Not only is this mixture good to have on hand for smoothies, oatmeal, and parfaits—it'll just look really pretty sitting in your fridge.
- **Muffins.** When they're not loaded with refined flour or sugar, these baked goods are perfect to grab as you head out the door. My go-to is the mini Banana Blueberry Muffins on page 99.
- **Beets.** Roast these root vegetables ahead of time so you can use them throughout the week as salad toppings, in vegetable wraps, or as an earthy side at lunch or dinner. See the

Roasted Beets recipe—it's one of my all-time favorites—on page 97.

· **Almond flour.** Sometimes it's hard to find or not readily stocked, and many stores charge quite a bit for this "specialty" item. Buy whole raw almonds and process the heck out of them. Boom, almond flour.

And these are the foods that, for me, often aren't worth prepping:

· **Corn.** Picture yourself shucking cob after cob to get those kernels for the Stuffed Quinoa Peppers (page 85) or any other recipe that calls for corn. Clearly not ideal for anyone who's short on time—so buy it bagged or canned.

· **Butternut squash.** Unless you're a master with unwieldy vegetables and sharp knives, cubed squash—found in Roasted Vegetable Hash with Fried Egg (page 76), Honey Roasted Butternut Squash (page 96), and Thai Salad (page 89)—is easier to buy pre-cubed.

· **Fish.** If I know a more-hectic-than-usual week is looming, I might grab pre-seasoned fish at the grocery store. One of my favorites is California garlic on tilapia.

· **Kale.** Buying a bag of chopped kale makes grabbing one serving—the standard is a handful—a no-brainer.

CHAPTER 7

Recipes for Every Meal

Now that you know the four clean eating habits—and understand why they're so important to your health—it's time to put them into action. Depending on where you started in this journey, you may only have to tweak a few of your favorite ingredients . . . or you may have to overhaul your entire diet. Either way, the resources you need to ease into a clean eating lifestyle are in this book.

Which brings us to the 4 × 4 recipes. All of these are designed to fit the four clean eating habits: the dinner options contain minimal starches, all are low in sugar and sodium, and none include alcohol. If it sounds like a lot to take in, you can rest assured that they're also easy to make—even if you're new or clumsy in the kitchen—and as flavorful as they are nutritious.

These recipes are what my family and I eat regularly; I'm basically dumping my recipe box onto the following pages. We're a motley crew of taste preferences and dietary needs, and we walk away from the dinner table full and happy. (My clients have started making many of these recipes, too.) I think you'll like these clean breakfast, lunch, dinner, sides, dessert, snack, and smoothie ideas as much as we all do.

4 × 4 BREAKFAST RECIPES

Roasted Vegetable Hash with Fried Egg

1 carrot, peeled
1 parsnip, peeled
6 mushrooms
½ onion, peeled
1 zucchini
1 yellow squash
1 butternut squash
1 sweet potato, peeled
2 tablespoons extra virgin olive oil
1 teaspoon ground cumin
1 teaspoon paprika
2 tablespoons minced garlic
1 whole egg
2 egg whites

Preheat the oven to 425°F. Cut all of the vegetables into bite-size pieces and mix with the olive oil, cumin, paprika, and garlic in a medium bowl. Spread the vegetables on a baking sheet and bake for 20 minutes. Remove from the oven. Fry 1 whole egg and 2 egg whites for each serving that you scoop from the batch of hash, and use as a topping.

Note: These vegetables happen to be my family's favorites—fill up the baking sheet with your favorites! Capitalize on whatever is in season, grab what's available in your fridge, or stick to what you know you love.

Whole-Wheat Crepes

3 eggs
⅔ cup skim milk or unsweetened almond milk
2 tablespoons melted unsalted butter or butter substitute
   (optional)
¼ teaspoon salt
⅓ cup whole-wheat flour

Beat the eggs, milk, butter (if using), and salt in a small bowl. Mix in the flour. For tastier crepes, cover the batter loosely and let sit either in the fridge or at room temperature for 30 to 60 minutes. Pour a heavy spoonful into a hot skillet, moving it side to side to spread the batter in a thin, even layer. Flip when it's slightly brown on the edges.

TOPPINGS:
Blueberry compote (see page 81)
Sliced bananas
Natural creamy peanut butter

FOR THE PEACH RASPBERRY COMPOTE:
1 pint raspberries
1 teaspoon arrowroot powder
1 tablespoon agave nectar
½ cup water
1 peach, peeled and diced (or ½ cup frozen peaches)
   Bring all ingredients to a boil, stirring continuously and smashing the peaches and berries as you go. Reduce the heat and simmer for 5 minutes. Refrigerate or use immediately.

Breakfast of Champions

5 fried egg whites
½ cup cooked old-fashioned oatmeal
5 or 6 strawberries
½ teaspoon brown sugar (optional)

Cut up the fried egg whites and mix with the oatmeal in a small bowl. Top with the berries and brown sugar (if using).

Apple Cinnamon Oatmeal Pecan Crunch

1 cup steel-cut oatmeal
2½ cups water
1½ cups unsweetened vanilla almond milk
1 cup chopped apple
1 tablespoon maple syrup/desired sweetener

1½ teaspoons ground cinnamon
½ teaspoon vanilla extract
1 handful of pecans

Spray the inside of a slow cooker with cooking spray and add all of the ingredients except the pecans. Cook on low overnight for about 9 hours (I start it at about 9 p.m. for a 6 a.m. breakfast). Top with pecans before serving.

> Note: Use your favorite nut as a topper—they'll all add that crunch factor!

Avocado Toast with Fried Egg

½ avocado
Sprinkle of sea salt
Squeeze of lemon
1 slice whole-wheat toast
2 slices tomato
1 whole egg and 1 egg white, fried (optional)

Mash up the avocado in a bowl with the salt and lemon juice. Spread on the toast and top with tomato slices. If desired, top with the fried eggs.

> Note: If you're craving toast in the evening, replace the whole-wheat bread with almond- or coconut-flour bread to reduce the amount of starchy carbs. (If you're going with store-bought options, find them in the freezer or refrigerated section.) These breads don't toast very well, so try heating them up in the oven or microwave to get that warm base.

Easy Yogurt Parfait

1 cup reduced-fat plain Greek yogurt
½ teaspoon vanilla extract
1 tablespoon natural peanut butter or PB2
½ teaspoon agave nectar or maple syrup
1 handful of fresh strawberries, blueberries, and/or raspberries
Reduced-sugar granola

Mix the yogurt, vanilla, peanut butter, and agave in a small bowl. Top with the berries and granola.

Veggie, Egg, and Quinoa Casserole

8 eggs
½ pound turkey breakfast sausage (optional)
1 cup diced red bell pepper
1 cup chopped onion
1 cup chopped mushrooms
½ cup chopped spinach
½ cup uncooked quinoa
1½ teaspoons minced garlic
1 cup unsweetened almond milk
¼ teaspoon salt
¼ teaspoon black pepper
1 cup Italian blend shredded cheese

Preheat the oven to 350°F. Mix all of the ingredients except the cheese in a medium bowl and pour into an 8 × 8-inch baking dish. Cover with foil and bake for 40 minutes, making sure it's cooked all the way through in the center. Uncover, spread the cheese on top, and place back in the oven until the cheese is melted.

Tour de Breakfast

Part I: The Omelette

1 whole egg
3 egg whites
½ teaspoon black pepper
1 teaspoon crushed red pepper flakes
½ piece 2 percent pepper jack cheese (pre-sliced)
¼ cup premade pepper mix (see page 73)
1 bell pepper (red, yellow, orange, or green)
3 jalapeño peppers
1 white onion

Beat the eggs, black pepper, and red pepper flakes in a small bowl, and pour the mixture evenly into a frying fan. As the eggs begin to firm up, add the cheese and the pepper mix. Use a spatula to ease around the edge of the omelet, then fold it in half and heat until both sides are golden brown.

Part II: The Oatmeal

½ cup old-fashioned oatmeal
½ teaspoon brown sugar
1 handful of blueberries, raspberries, and strawberries

Cook the oatmeal, then top with brown sugar and berries.

Part III: Side of turkey sausage (optional)

Sautéed Spinach and Scrambled Egg Burrito for Two

2 whole eggs
2 egg whites
½ garlic clove, minced
Salt and pepper to taste
Pinch of crushed red pepper flakes
2 handfuls of spinach
2 whole-wheat tortillas
¼ cup cooked and drained turkey sausage
¼ avocado
2 tablespoons salsa

Scramble the eggs with the garlic, salt, pepper, and red pepper flakes. Add the spinach when the eggs are nearly done. Warm up the tortillas. Wrap the scrambled eggs in each tortilla and top each with half of the avocado and half of the salsa.

Lemon Pancakes with Blueberry Compote

FOR THE LEMON PANCAKES:
3 cups almond flour
1½ cups unsweetened almond milk

½ teaspoon baking soda
3 eggs
1 teaspoon lemon zest
1 teaspoon lemon juice

FOR THE BLUEBERRY COMPOTE:
1 pint blueberries
1 tablespoon agave nectar
1 teaspoon arrowroot powder
½ cup water

To make the pancakes: Mix all of the ingredients in a medium bowl. Spray a skillet with cooking spray and make sure it is hot for your first batch. Drop in a large spoonful of batter and cook until you see bubbles forming. Flip and do the same on the other side.

To make the compote: Bring all of the ingredients to a boil, stirring continuously and smashing the blueberries as you go. Reduce the heat and simmer for 5 minutes. Refrigerate or use immediately.

To serve: Top the pancakes with blueberry compote.

---

4 × 4 LUNCH RECIPES

Root Vegetable Tacos

2 corn tortillas
Roasted Vegetable Hash (see page 76)
1 avocado, sliced

FOR THE CHIPOTLE AIOLI:
1 chipotle pepper, chopped
½ cup light mayo or vegan mayo (like Vegenaise)
1 tablespoon adobo sauce

To make the aioli: Put the ingredients in a bowl and mix thoroughly.

To make the tacos: Fill the corn tortillas with the vegetable hash. Top with avocado slices. Drizzle chipotle aioli over top.

Hummus Sandwich

2 tablespoons red pepper hummus
2 slices Ezekiel bread
½ avocado, sliced
2 thin tomato slices
¼ cup alfalfa sprouts
Sliced red onions

Spread hummus on each slice of Ezekiel bread and add all of the other ingredients to assemble the sandwich.

Apple Cider Salad

2 cups mixed greens
1 apple, cored and chopped
4 ounces crumbled blue cheese
Shredded rotisserie chicken (optional)
Black pepper to taste

FOR THE MAPLE PECANS:
½ cup pecan pieces
Pinch of salt
2 teaspoons maple syrup

Add the pecans and salt to a skillet over medium-high heat, and cook until brown. Add the maple syrup and reduce the heat to medium. Let the syrup mix in, then remove from the heat.

FOR THE APPLE CIDER VINAIGRETTE:
2 tablespoons Bragg's Apple Cider Vinegar
2 tablespoons extra virgin olive oil
1 teaspoon minced garlic
¼ teaspoon onion powder
¼ teaspoon oregano
Pinch of salt and pepper
¼ teaspoon onion powder

Combine vinaigrette ingredients and stir together, then drizzle over salad and toss.

Kale Quinoa Asian Salad

1 cup cooked quinoa
2 cups chopped kale
½ cup shredded carrot
½ cup toasted almonds
1 cup halved cherry tomatoes
½ cup currants

FOR THE ASIAN VINAIGRETTE:
2 tablespoons extra virgin olive oil
2 tablespoons rice vinegar (or balsamic, based on taste)
1 tablespoon low-sodium soy sauce
1 teaspoon minced garlic
1 teaspoon honey
1 teaspoon shaved fresh ginger
½ teaspoon sesame oil
1 tablespoon water

While the quinoa is cooking, prepare the dressing by combining all the ingredients and mixing them thoroughly. Pour 2 tablespoons of dressing on the chopped kale to let it soak in and set aside. Once the quinoa is cooled, mix all ingredients in a medium bowl.

Rice Paper Wraps

2 rice papers (they're about the size of a tortilla)
½ avocado, thinly sliced
1 handful of broccoli slaw
2 pinches of chopped fresh cilantro
½ red bell pepper, thinly sliced
½ carrot, shaved
¼ cucumber, seeded and sliced lengthwise
1 cup shredded cooked chicken (optional)
Annie Chun's Thai Peanut Sauce

Fill a plate with water and dip each rice paper wrap in it for about 5 seconds, then let dry on a paper towel. Mix all of the ingredients in a small bowl, place half in the in the center of each wrap, and roll them up. Serve with peanut sauce for dipping.

Spicy Bahn Mi Wrap

  2 grilled chicken tenders
  1 whole-wheat wrap
  1 handful of spinach
  Fresh basil

  FOR THE CHICKEN MARINADE:
  1 tablespoon Sriracha
  1 tablespoon honey
  ¼ cup water
  1 garlic clove, minced
  1 teaspoon minced fresh ginger

Mix the marinade ingredients in a small bowl and pour over the chicken tenders in a freezer bag. Let rest for 30 to 45 minutes.

  FOR THE SRIRACHA DRESSING:
  1 tablespoon Sriracha
  ¼ cup plain Greek yogurt
    Mix the dressing ingredients in a small bowl and set aside.

  FOR THE PICKLED ONION:
  ½ onion, thinly sliced
  2 tablespoons rice vinegar
  1½ teaspoon stevia
    Mix the ingredients in a small bowl, cover, and place in the refrigerator.

Assemble by spreading the Sriracha dressing on the warmed wrap, then add both chicken tenders. Sprinkle pickled onions, spinach, and a couple of basil leaves on top, then roll up.

Chicken Salad

2 pulled boneless chicken breasts, grilled, boiled, or baked
¼ cup Greek yogurt
⅓ cup chopped celery
2 shallots, chopped
⅓ cup halved grapes
1 whole-wheat sandwich thin or a bed of greens

FOR THE TOASTED WALNUTS:

Fill a small skillet with walnuts and heat over medium-high heat. Sprinkle with salt to taste and cook, tossing until they are brown.

Mix the chicken and yogurt thoroughly in a small bowl. Blend in the celery, shallots, and grapes and spread on a whole-wheat sandwich thin or over a bed of greens.

Note: You can also use pulled-apart rotisserie chicken—just make sure to remove its high-fat skin first.

Stuffed Quinoa Peppers

½ pound light ground beef or turkey (optional)
1½ cups cooked quinoa
½ pack salt-free taco seasoning
6 red bell peppers, halved and seeded
¾ cup low-sodium black beans, drained and rinsed
½ cup finely chopped fresh cilantro
1 cup corn kernels
1 teaspoon garlic powder
1 can green chiles
½ teaspoon onion powder
1 cup diced cherry tomatoes
¼ cup light or fat-free feta cheese
½ cup shredded pepper jack cheese

Preheat the oven to 425°F. If using beef or turkey, cook it with the taco seasoning. If leaving the beef out, then mix the taco seasoning in with the cooked quinoa. Place the bell pepper halves on a foil-lined baking sheet with the cut side down. Spray the peppers with olive oil (either from a sprayer or a store-bought can) and roast for about 10 minutes. Mix the beef or turkey (if using), quinoa, beans, cilantro, corn, garlic powder, chiles, onion powder, tomatoes, and feta in a large bowl. Flip the peppers, cut side up, and fill with the quinoa mixture. Place back in the oven for another 10 minutes and sprinkle the pepper jack on top for the last minute or so, until melted.

Quinoa Tabouli Salad

1 cup cooked quinoa
3 tablespoons extra virgin olive oil
3 tablespoons lemon juice
½ teaspoon sea salt
1 cup chopped fresh parsley
½ bunch chopped fresh cilantro
3 tomatoes, diced
2 scallions, white and green parts, thinly sliced
¼ cup chopped cucumber
¼ cup reduced-sugar dried cranberries

Mix all of the ingredients in a large bowl and refrigerate until ready to serve.

---

4 × 4 DINNER RECIPES

Stir-Fry with Cauliflower Rice

FOR THE CAULIFLOWER RICE:
1 head cauliflower, chopped
Extra virgin olive oil
Salt and pepper

Put the cauliflower in a food processor and chop until the pieces are roughly the size of rice grains. Place a tablespoon of olive oil in a skillet over medium-high heat and add the cauliflower after the oil is hot. Add a pinch of salt and pepper and cook for 5 to 10 minutes or until soft.

FOR THE STIR-FRY SAUCE:

2 tablespoons vegetable oil
2 garlic cloves, minced (or 2 tablespoons minced garlic)
¼ cup low-sodium soy sauce
¼ cup water
3 tablespoons honey
2 tablespoons corn starch

> Heat the oil in a skillet and mix in the rest of the ingredients, letting the sauce cook for a few minutes.

1 pound chicken breast, cut into pieces (optional)
1 red bell pepper, sliced
1 onion, sliced
1 broccoli crown, cut into florets

Put the chicken into the skillet with half of the stir-fry sauce. Cook for 5 minutes, then add the bell pepper, onion, broccoli, and the rest of the sauce and continue cooking until the chicken is done. Place a serving of the stir-fry over a scoop of cauliflower rice.

Chicken Tenders (Traditional Flavor)

1 cup almond flour
1 teaspoon garlic powder
½ teaspoon salt
½ teaspoon black pepper
½ teaspoon cayenne pepper (optional)
2 egg whites
2 pounds chicken tenders

Preheat the oven to 450°F. Mix the almond flour, garlic powder, salt, black pepper, and cayenne pepper (if using) in a small bowl and pour the mixture onto a plate. Put the egg whites in a nearby bowl. Dip the chicken tenders in the egg whites, then evenly coat them in the flour mixture and lay out on a cookie sheet sprayed with cooking spray. Bake for about 16 minutes, flipping them halfway through, until both sides are crisp.

Chicken Tenders (Italian Blend)

    1 cup almond flour
    ½ teaspoon salt
    ½ teaspoon pepper
    1 tablespoon Italian-blend seasoning
    1 teaspoon garlic powder
    3 egg whites
    2 pounds chicken tenders
    Italian-blend cheese
    Low-sodium spaghetti sauce

Preheat the oven to 450°F. Mix the almond flour, salt, pepper, Italian seasoning, and garlic powder in a small bowl and pour the mixture onto a plate. Put the egg whites in a nearby bowl. Dip the chicken tenders in the egg whites, then evenly coat them in the flour mixture and lay out on a cookie sheet sprayed with cooking spray. Bake for about 16 minutes, flipping them halfway through, until both sides are crisp. Lightly coat the top of the tenders with the cheese and, if needed, place back in the oven to melt it. Serve with spaghetti sauce for dipping.

Lasagna Spaghetti Squash Casserole

    2 spaghetti squash
    2 cups low-sodium or reduced-sugar spaghetti sauce
    1 pound ground beef, cooked (optional)
    1½ cups light ricotta cheese
    1 cup shredded mozzarella
    2 tablespoons chopped fresh parsley

Preheat the oven to 375°F. Perforate each squash with a fork and bake for 1 hour. Once cool, cut each squash in half lengthwise and scoop out the fleshy middle containing the seeds. (Use a serrated knife for the best results.) Then use a fork to scrape out the squash, creating strips like spaghetti as you do so.

Place 1 cup of spaghetti sauce on the bottom of an 8 × 8-inch baking dish. Spread the spaghetti squash evenly as the next layer.

The next layer is the beef (if using). Then spread a layer of ricotta cheese. The next layer is the rest of the sauce. Top with the mozzarella, then sprinkle the parsley on top. Cover the dish with foil and bake for 15 to 20 minutes, until the cheese is melted. Uncover and cook for another 5 minutes.

Sautéed Brussels Sprouts with Fried Egg

½ bag shaved Brussels sprouts (or shave your own)
¼ teaspoon cayenne pepper
½ tablespoon garlic powder
Salt to taste
1 whole egg
2 egg whites
1 small handful of sautéed almonds

Spray a skillet with cooking spray, add the Brussels sprouts, and cook over medium-high heat. Mix in the cayenne pepper, garlic powder, and salt and let cook until the sprouts start turning brown. (Keep stirring until they are all brown and slightly crispy.) Place the egg whites into a separate skillet, and crack the whole egg on top, making sure not to burst the yolk. Let it fry, removing it from the heat before the yolk hardens—this includes one very careful flip of the eggs so as to not bust open the yolk. Quickly cook the other side, creating the runny yolk in the middle of all the egg whites. Place the Brussels sprouts on a plate and top with the fried eggs. Sprinkle the sautéed almonds over everything.

Thai Salad

FOR THE SALAD BASE:
1 carrot, peeled
1 red bell pepper, cored, seeded, and sliced or diced
1 green bell pepper, cored, seeded, and sliced or diced
½ jicama
1 red onion

1 zucchini
1 yellow squash
Pinch of chopped fresh basil
½ bag broccoli slaw
½ avocado, thinly sliced

Note: Add or swap in your other favorite vegetables for an extra-colorful mix.

FOR THE DRESSING:
2 tablespoons low-sodium soy sauce or coconut aminos
1½ teaspoons fish sauce
2 tablespoons rice vinegar (unseasoned)
Dash of Sriracha (or hot sauce of choice)
1 teaspoon minced fresh ginger
2 garlic cloves, minced
1 teaspoon agave nectar
1 teaspoon sesame oil
1 tablespoon extra virgin olive oil

Note: Be frugal with the fish sauce, as it is high in sodium and intense in flavor. A little goes a long way!

Use a food processor to julienne the carrot, bell peppers, jicama, onion, zucchini, and yellow squash. Place in a large salad bowl. Tear the basil leaves and add to the salad, along with the broccoli slaw. Then mix all of the dressing ingredients except the oils in a small bowl. Slowly add the oils, whisking as you incorporate them into the other ingredients. Pour the dressing over the salad and mix well. Add the sliced avocado on top.

Note: This is a very small amount of dressing for the volume of the salad, so let it marinate for about 30 minutes before serving. Mix it up three or four times while you are waiting to eat.

Note: Although this salad can be a meal by itself, you can easily add grilled tilapia, grilled chicken breast, or Asian tuna steak (recipe follows) to provide a protein.

Asian Tuna Steak on a Bed of Sautéed Kale

2 6-ounce tuna steaks
1 teaspoon extra virgin olive oil
2 large handfuls of kale
2 tablespoons water
¼ teaspoon salt
2 teaspoons minced garlic
Spoonful of gari (pickled ginger, optional)

FOR THE MARINADE:
2 tablespoons coconut aminos
1 tablespoon sesame oil
2 garlic cloves, minced
1 teaspoon ground or minced fresh ginger

Mix the marinade ingredients in a small bowl. Place the tuna steaks in a resealable plastic bag and top with the marinade. Let the fish rest in the refrigerator for 30 minutes, flipping the bag once halfway through. Remove the tuna from the bag, set aside the marinade, and grill the tuna for 3 to 4 minutes on each side. Brush with reserved marinade if desired. While the fish is cooking, heat the olive oil in a skillet, add the kale, and sauté. When the kale is tender, add the water, salt, and garlic. Cook, covered, over medium-low heat for 10 to 15 minutes, stirring occasionally. The kale should be fully tender when it's done. If desired, serve with a spoonful of gari.

> Note: The grilling time will vary according to the thickness of the fish steaks. Tuna dries out if it's overcooked, so keep in mind that less is more—and that rare tuna is delicious!

Scallop Spinach Salad with Bacon

FOR THE SALAD:
1 onion
1 teaspoon extra virgin olive oil
6 tablespoons grated Parmesan cheese
6 sea scallops

Salt and pepper to taste
3 slices bacon
1 bunch of spinach

FOR THE DRESSING:
3 tablespoons good-quality balsamic vinegar
1 teaspoon maple syrup
2 garlic cloves, minced
2 tablespoons extra virgin olive oil

> Mix the dressing ingredients in a small bowl, adding the oil last, and set aside.

Begin by caramelizing the onion, since this will take a while. Slice the onion to the desired thickness (making ⅛-inch slices will prevent them from drying out) and toss with the olive oil in a small bowl. Place in a frying pan over low heat and allow the onion to caramelize for approximately 40 minutes, stirring occasionally.

Preheat the oven to 350°F. Put a piece of parchment paper on a cookie sheet, top with 6 mounds of grated Parmesan cheese (1 tablespoon for each scallop) and bake until golden brown. Watch closely because it only takes about 5 minutes for these to crisp up! Take the Parmesan crisps out of the oven and set aside.

> Note: You can caramelize the onions and make the Parmesan crisps the day before—just store in airtight containers overnight. You can use these for other salads as well.

Reduce the oven to 250°F. Lay the scallops on paper towels, add salt and pepper to taste, and allow to dry thoroughly. While the scallops are drying, cut the bacon into small pieces and crisp them in a frying pan over medium heat. When the bacon is crisp, set it on paper towels to drain. Drain all but 1 teaspoon of the bacon grease from the frying pan and return to the burner over medium heat. When the pan is screaming hot, place the scallops in the pan and sear on both sides until golden brown. Place the scallops in an ovenproof pan (or keep them in an ovenproof frying pan) and place them in the oven for about 6 minutes while you assemble the remainder of the salad.

Place the dressing in the bottom of a large salad bowl and top with the spinach, Parmesan crisps, crumbled bacon, and caramelized onions. Toss the salad with the dressing and top with the cooked scallops.

Zucchini Noodles with Pesto and Tilapia

2 medium zucchini
Grated Parmesan cheese
Tilapia or other fish of your choice

FOR THE PESTO:
1 bunch fresh basil leaves
½ cup toasted pine nuts
½ cup grated Parmesan cheese
2 garlic cloves (or 2 tablespoons minced garlic)
¾ cup extra virgin olive oil
    Blend all of the pesto ingredients in a food processor.

Use a spiralizer to cut the zucchini into spaghetti-like strips. Place the zucchini noodles in a skillet and warm up over medium heat for a couple of minutes. Top with grated Parmesan and 2 tablespoons of the pesto. Mix well. Serve topped with grilled fish.

Note: Pour any remaining pesto into ice cube trays and freeze. Warm up the amount you need whenever you want it for another recipe. You can also save time by using oven-ready fish from the grocery store and/or low-sodium store-bought pesto sauce.

Lemon Pepper Cod

2 cod fillets (I prefer the thick end of the fillet)
1 teaspoon extra virgin olive oil
Zest and juice of 1 lemon
Lemon pepper seasoning (Trader Joe's makes a good one)

Dry the cod fillets and rub them with olive oil. Top the fillets with the lemon zest and sprinkle with lemon pepper seasoning as desired. Let the fillets rest in the refrigerator for 15 minutes and then grill for 3 minutes. Top with fresh lemon juice.

> Note: This is one of the world's easiest dinners! Two great side options: grilled asparagus and kale salad.

Chicken Caprese

2 chicken breasts
Garlic powder
2 ounces fresh mozzarella cheese
1 tomato, sliced
2 teaspoons balsamic vinegar
Fresh basil
Black pepper to taste

Preheat the oven to 350°F. Lightly season the chicken with garlic powder and grill or bake thoroughly. Put 1 ounce of mozzarella on top of each chicken breast and bake for a couple minutes, removing from the oven before the cheese is fully melted. Top each breast with 2 tomato slices, drizzle with balsamic vinegar, and sprinkle with basil leaves. Top with fresh black pepper.

Kale Salad with Chicken

4 ounces cooked and pulled chicken
1 handful of chopped romaine
2 handfuls of chopped kale
1 handful of Oil-Free Sautéed Almonds (see page 98)
¼ teaspoon cayenne pepper
½ teaspoon garlic powder

FOR THE DRESSING:
2 tablespoons balsamic vinegar
2 tablespoons extra virgin olive oil
2 tablespoons water
1 teaspoon minced garlic
1 teaspoon maple syrup

¼ teaspoon onion powder
¼ teaspoon oregano
Pinch of salt and pepper

Combine all dressing ingredients and mix thoroughly.

Warm up the chicken in a skillet. Place the romaine in a salad bowl. Process the kale into really small pieces in a food processor, then add it to the romaine. Add the rest of the salad ingredients and toss with 2 tablespoons of the dressing.

Lettuce Wrap Tacos

1 pound lean ground beef (preferably 97 percent lean)
½ to ⅓ package low-sodium taco seasoning
Bibb lettuce

TOPPINGS:
Sliced avocado
Light or fat-free sour cream
2 percent shredded Mexican-blend cheese
Salsa
Diced tomatoes
Diced jalapeño peppers
Chopped fresh cilantro
Premade pepper mix (see page 73)

Brown the beef and drain. Add the taco seasoning with water, following the directions on the package. Grab a big leaf of Bibb lettuce and fill with the seasoned beef. Fill up the lettuce with your favorite toppings, then roll up the lettuce.

4 × 4 SIDE RECIPES

Roasted Broccoli with Parmesan Cheese

1 head broccoli, chopped
2 teaspoons extra virgin olive oil
1 teaspoon minced garlic
Salt and pepper to taste
½ lemon
¼ cup shredded Parmesan cheese

Preheat the oven to 400°F. Toss the broccoli, olive oil, and garlic in a medium bowl. Spread the broccoli evenly on a baking sheet and sprinkle lightly with salt and pepper. Bake for 15 to 20 minutes. Remove from the oven and squeeze the lemon lightly on top, then sprinkle with Parmesan. Place the baking sheet back in the oven to melt the cheese.

Mashed Cauliflower

1 head cauliflower
¼ cup unsweetened almond milk or skim milk
½ teaspoon garlic powder or minced garlic
Salt and pepper to taste

Chop the cauliflower and steam it until soft. Place the cauliflower, milk, and garlic in a food processor and blend until it has the consistency of mashed potatoes. Add salt and pepper to taste.

Honey Roasted Butternut Squash

1 pound butternut squash, peeled and cubed
1 tablespoon extra virgin olive oil
1½ tablespoons honey
Pinch of salt and pepper
1 handful of chopped pecans

Preheat the oven to 400°F. Toss the squash, olive oil, honey, salt, and pepper in a medium bowl. Spread the squash evenly on a baking sheet sprayed with cooking spray. Bake for 35 to 45 minutes, until the squash is soft and browned. Top with chopped pecans.

Note: To save time, buy peeled and cubed butternut squash in the fresh food section of the grocery store.

Roasted Asparagus

1 bunch asparagus
1½ tablespoons extra virgin olive oil
1 tablespoon minced garlic
Salt and pepper to taste
2 tablespoons balsamic vinegar

Preheat the oven to 400°F. Snap the woody ends off the asparagus and spread out on a baking sheet. Coat in olive oil and garlic, and sprinkle with salt and pepper. Drizzle the balsamic vinegar over the asparagus, then bake for about 15 minutes.

Roasted Beets

3 medium beets
1 small package chopped walnuts
Pinch of salt
1 teaspoon extra virgin olive oil
1 ounce goat cheese

Preheat the oven to 425°F. Cut the tops and bottoms off the beets and wrap each one in foil. Place on a baking sheet and bake for 45 to 60 minutes. While they bake, toast the walnuts: place the walnuts in a small skillet over medium-high heat, sprinkle with salt, and cook until they are brown. (Keep an eye on them, as they go from brown to burned quickly!) When the beets are done, let cool, unwrap, and place under cold water to slip the skin off easily. Dice the beets and toss them with olive oil in a medium bowl. Combine the beets with crumbled goat cheese and walnuts.

Simply Roasted Brussels Sprouts

2 tablespoons sesame oil
1 bag Brussels sprouts, halved
1 tablespoon warm water
1 tablespoon light soy sauce
1 tablespoon honey
1 tablespoon minced garlic
½ onion, thinly sliced
¼ teaspoon crushed red pepper flakes

Heat the sesame oil in a skillet for 5 minutes over medium-high heat. Place the Brussels sprouts in a single layer, each half face down, on the hot skillet and cook without stirring for 4 minutes, or until brown. Continue cooking and stirring for the next few minutes. Mix the rest of the ingredients in a small bowl while the sprouts are cooking. Pour the sauce over the sprouts in the pan and heat until warm.

Note: Not stirring the sprouts at first is key! This makes for much crispier and tastier sprouts.

4 × 4 SNACK RECIPES

Oil-Free Sautéed Almonds

1 6-ounce bag sliced almonds
⅛ teaspoon salt
1½ tablespoons maple syrup

Cook just the almonds in a skillet over medium-high heat until slightly brown. Stir in the salt and cook until the almonds are fully brown. Stir in the maple syrup—and keep stirring, as it will start to bubble and can burn quickly. Pour the almonds on a plate to cool.

Note: This recipe also works with chopped pecans.

Note: Add ½ teaspoon cayenne pepper for some kick—or a lot more for a real punch.

Oven-Roasted Spicy Almonds

1 6-ounce bag sliced almonds
1 egg white
1 tablespoon honey
1 tablespoon light brown sugar
½ tablespoon cayenne pepper

Preheat the oven to 425°F. Mix all of the ingredients in a small bowl. Spray a baking sheet with cooking spray and spread the coated almonds evenly over the sheet. Bake for 8 to 10 minutes. When golden brown, flip all of the almonds and return to the oven to brown the other side. Let the almonds cool and break them apart for easy storage and snacking.

Note: These burn easily, so keep a watchful eye on the baking sheet.

Banana Blueberry Muffins

3 super-ripe bananas
2 tablespoons melted coconut oil
3 tablespoons maple syrup
½ teaspoon baking powder
½ teaspoon baking soda
1½ cups almond flour
1 small package blueberries

Preheat the oven to 375°F. Mash the bananas in a medium bowl, then mix in the rest of the ingredients except the blueberries. Fold in the blueberries. Spray a mini muffin tin with cooking spray and fill each cup ¾ full. Bake for 15 minutes.

Note: These mini muffins are a great, filling on-the-go snack—just toss one or two in an airtight plastic bag.

Whole-Wheat Banana Wrap

Natural creamy peanut butter
1 whole-wheat wrap
1 banana
Reduced-sugar granola

Spread the peanut butter on the wrap. Slice the banana and spread a handful of slices on the wrap. Sprinkle the granola on top. Roll up the tortilla and slice into bite-sized pieces.

Note: Swap in diced apple instead of the banana for a crunchier snack. Or use both!

Classic Veggies and Dip

VEGGIES:
Broccoli florets
Sliced bell peppers (red, orange, and yellow are my favorites)
Mushrooms
Sugar snap peas
Cauliflower
Cucumbers
Jalapeño peppers, seeded

DIPS:
Hummus
Greek yogurt veggie dip

Note: Watch the amount of carbs if you opt for store-bought hummus—this is to be munched on before evening.

Note: Thanks to Prep Day, this snack will be waiting for you in the fridge.

Not-So-Boring Brown Rice Cake

1 brown rice cake
2 tablespoons natural peanut butter
Honey or fresh berries

Spread the peanut butter on the rice cake and drizzle with honey or top with berries.

Peanut Butter Apple Crunch

    1 apple
    Natural peanut butter
    Reduced-sugar granola

Quarter the apple and scoop out the center of each piece, replacing it with your favorite natural peanut butter. Sprinkle granola on top of each piece.

---

4 × 4 DESSERT RECIPES

Note: These desserts are an incredibly wicked combination of nutritious and delicious. But that doesn't mean you should overindulge— you're still only eating one serving at a time.

Almond Butter No-Bake Bar with Berries

    1 cup creamy almond butter
    2 tablespoons melted coconut oil
    ¼ teaspoon vanilla extract
    Pinch of salt
    Strawberries or blueberries

Mix the almond butter, coconut oil, vanilla, and salt in a small bowl. Spread the mixture in an 8 × 8-inch pan lined with parchment paper. Place the pan in the freezer until the mixture is firm. Slice into about 16 bars and top each piece with berries before serving.

Cookie Dough Hummus

1 15-ounce can chickpeas, drained and rinsed
½ teaspoon vanilla extract
¼ cup old-fashioned oatmeal
Pinch of salt
¼ cup natural creamy peanut butter
¼ cup unsweetened vanilla almond milk
1½ tablespoons brown sugar (or sweetener of choice)
⅓ cup dark chocolate chips

Blend all of the ingredients except the chocolate chips in a food processor—be prepared to blend for quite a while. (You may need to add more almond milk to get the consistency of hummus.) Pour into a serving dish and mix in the chocolate chips. Serve with graham crackers or just a spoon!

Peanut Butter Chocolate Protein Brownies

½ cup almond or whole-wheat flour
2 whole eggs
3 egg whites
3 tablespoons unsweetened almond milk
½ cup natural peanut butter
4 tablespoons PB2
1 scoop chocolate protein powder
¼ cup stevia (or sweetener of choice)
½ cup unsweetened applesauce
2 teaspoons vanilla extract
½ teaspoon baking powder
½ teaspoon salt
¾ cup dark chocolate chips

Preheat the oven to 350°F. Mix all of the ingredients except the chocolate chips in a large bowl. Fold in the chocolate chips and spoon the mixture into an 8 × 8-inch baking pan sprayed with cooking spray. Bake for about 20 minutes or until the center is cooked all the way through. Cut into 2-inch squares.

No-Bake Individual Cheesecakes

FOR THE BASE:
½ cup dates
½ cup raw almonds
1 teaspoon vanilla extract
1 tablespoon water

FOR THE FILLING:
¼ cup fat-free cream cheese
¼ cup plain Greek yogurt
1 tablespoon agave nectar
1 teaspoon stevia

FOR THE TOPPING:
2 tablespoons plain Greek yogurt
2 teaspoons ground cinnamon
2 teaspoons stevia

Spray the cups of a mini muffin pan with cooking spray. Use a food processor to blend the dates, almonds, vanilla, and water until the mixture becomes sticky and doughlike. Smush it into each muffin cup to create the bottom of each mini cheesecake. Now mix the filling ingredients together in the food processor until well blended, and evenly distribute this mixture on top of the base layer. Lastly, mix the topping ingredients in a bowl and then put a dollop on top of each mini cheesecake bite. Freeze until firm.

Note: Using a 24-cup mini muffin tin practically requires portion control.

Two-Layer Peanut Butter Brownies

FOR THE BOTTOM LAYER:
1 cup peanuts
1 cup dates or figs
1 tablespoons cocoa
¼ cup dark chocolate chips

FOR THE TOP LAYER:

¾ cup natural peanut butter

3½ tablespoons maple syrup

1 tablespoon melted coconut oil

2 tablespoons unsweetened vanilla almond milk (more if you need it to be more spreadable)

Pinch of sea salt (⅛ teaspoon)

Spray an 8 × 8-inch baking pan with cooking spray. Mix the bottom-layer ingredients in a food processor, adding up to 2 tablespoons water, if needed, to make it a doughy consistency. Spread the mixture into the bottom of the pan; it will take some pressing and kneading to get it even all around. Then mix the top-layer ingredients in the food processor and spread that mixture on top of the base with a knife or your fingers. Freeze, cut into about 16 squares, and serve.

Note: You can change up the recipe by using other nuts, such as almonds or walnuts.

---

4 × 4 SMOOTHIE RECIPES

Berry Creme Smoothie

½ avocado

2 tablespoons old-fashioned oats

½ cup reduced-sugar vanilla Greek yogurt

5 strawberries

2 handfuls of blueberries

Splash of unsweetened almond milk

1 cup ice

Blend all ingredients until smooth.

Client Classic Smoothie

¾ cup unsweetened vanilla almond milk
2 cups ice
1 scoop vanilla protein powder
1 tablespoon cocoa powder
½ frozen banana
1 to 2 tablespoons natural peanut butter or PB2

Blend all ingredients until smooth.

Sweet Green Smoothie (2 servings)

2 cups unsweetened almond milk
1 scoop vanilla protein powder
2 handfuls of spinach or kale
1 tablespoon ground flax seed
1 cup frozen berries or mango
½ frozen banana

Blend all ingredients until smooth.

Green Apple Cinnamon Smoothie

1½ cups unsweetened almond milk
½ cup reduced-sugar vanilla Greek yogurt
1 handful of kale
1½ cups diced apple
1 tablespoon chia seeds
1 teaspoon ground cinnamon
1 teaspoon agave nectar or honey

Blend all ingredients until smooth.

Note: The apples don't have to be green—the kale gives this high-fiber smoothie its name!

Smooth Peachiness

½ cup old-fashioned oats
1½ cups frozen peaches
1 cup reduced-sugar vanilla Greek yogurt
½ cup unsweetened almond milk
1 tablespoon honey or agave nectar
¼ teaspoon vanilla extract
½ teaspoon ground cinnamon

Blend the oats into a powder, then add the rest of the ingredients. Continue to blend until smooth.

CHAPTER 8

Recipe Variations and Substitutions

Are you getting the most out of your baking ingredients? Here's one way to find out: picture yourself canvassing the grocery store as you load up your shopping cart. Most of us simply grab our go-to items from the shelves, check them off our list, and head for the checkout line.

Now I want you to take a closer look at that shopping list, especially at the items you've been buying for years, the ones that you use in the kitchen on a weekly—and sometimes daily—basis. Do they include all-purpose flour? A gallon of cow's milk? Sugar? Butter? These are staples in many, many recipes, and often feel as familiar as your oldest friends. But are these foods serving as high-grade fuel for your body? When you examine their nutritional content, are they the best choices you could be making? Are they doing their job?

The short answer to all of those questions: very possibly, no.

Some of these basic ingredients are actually bad for you, meaning they can deteriorate your health (*cough*, refined sugar, *cough*). Some are okay in small amounts, like butter. And some aren't unhealthy per se, but sitting just a few store shelves away are alternatives that will nourish your body with even more nutrients—like almond milk.

You may think I'm about to launch into a lecture. But where's the fun in that? Instead, I want you to think of this as an opportunity to get creative in the kitchen. Switching out ingredients for healthier options can be an ongoing game: once you figure out a way to make a standard recipe a bit healthier, make that your new baseline. Then take the tweaked recipe and try to make *that* one healthier. Years ago, I took my parents' pancake recipe, which used all-purpose flour, and incorporated some whole-wheat flour. That got the thumbs-up from my husband and kids—it tasted different, but not in a bad way. Then after a while, I began using all whole-wheat flour. That became the new normal for my family until a few years later, when we began experimenting with almond flour. I started out using store-bought almond flour, but it is a specialty item and a bit expensive—so making it from scratch became a new part of Prep Day. Constantly changing up the ingredients like this, making them higher in certain nutrients and different in taste, keeps both the chef and the hungry mouths entertained. I've spent years playing around with food modifications and substitutions, like a chemist honing her formulas in her lab, and I'll still be experimenting for years to come.

You likely use at least some of the following ingredients frequently, without even thinking about what they're adding to the recipe other than a particular taste or texture. So roll up your sleeves and experiment with these suggested modifications and variations. Get covered in almond dust and sticky maple syrup. Your meals will become better for you—and you can have more fun while you're at it.

THE INGREDIENT: All-Purpose Flour

In a way, you have to hand it to all-purpose flour. It's been used for thousands and thousands of years and is found in cuisines around the globe—despite the fact that it lacks a substantial amount of nutrients. All-purpose flour, which you'll also find labeled as white, occident, or refined flour, is extremely low in fiber compared to other varieties: a half cup of white flour contains about 1.5 grams of fiber, while that same amount of whole-wheat flour contains about 7.5 grams. (To their credit, some manufacturers do fortify their all-purpose flour with calcium and vitamin A or D to make up for what's lost in the refining process.)

Traditional thinking says you can't bake foods like bread, biscuits, cookies, and cakes without flour. But who says the *flour* has to be traditional? Next time you're in the baking aisle, look around at the diversity it offers in the form of alternatives to all-purpose flour. These are a few of my favorites.

The Substitutions:

100 percent whole-wheat flour

As its name implies, whole-wheat flour is derived from the complete wheat kernel—including parts called the bran and germ, which are processed out of regular flour. Retaining the bran and germ is a good thing, because they contain macronutrients like fiber (nearly four times as much!) and protein; you'll also get sizable doses of calcium, magnesium, zinc, and the antioxidant selenium, which plays a key role in your metabolism. Whole-wheat flour has a slightly nutty flavor as well as a denser texture that may take a while to get used to.

How to use it: Because of its unique flavor and texture, whole-wheat flour is best used in hearty breads rather than delicate pastries. If you're whipping up sturdier baked goods, swap out anywhere from 50 to 100 percent of the all-purpose flour for whole-wheat flour. If you want to try it with more delicate recipes, like pastries, replace up to 50 percent of the all-purpose flour with a whole-wheat pastry flour. For a milder taste and lighter-colored baked goods, look for white whole-wheat flour, which is made from hulled white spring wheat.

Try it in: Banana bread, blueberry or apple-cinnamon muffins, chocolate chip cookies, pitas, pizza dough

Almond flour

Made from blanched almonds, this version of flour will shower your body with protein, manganese, and vitamin E. It's also low in carbohydrates and sugar, meaning you can eat it later in the day. Almonds can lower your risk of cardiometabolic diseases, like heart disease, diabetes, and stroke.

How to use it: When baking with yeast, you can't use almond flour exactly like wheat flour—its gluten-free properties will restrict the dough from rising. The general rule is to replace 25 percent of a recipe's called-for flour with almond flour.

Try it in: Pancakes, muffins, dessert fillings, breading (see the pair of Chicken Tenders recipes on pages 87 and 88)

Coconut flour

Like almond flour, coconut flour is low in carbs, high in protein and fiber, and gluten free. Additionally, it's high in manganese and healthy fats, which your body uses as energy. It's made from dried coconut meat, so if you love the taste of coconut, you'll love infusing this flour into all sorts of recipes.

How to use it: For every cup of wheat flour, substitute ¼ cup to ⅓ cup of coconut flour. Because of its density and dryness, you'll also need to use more eggs, which act as a binder—for every cup of coconut flour you use, add six beaten eggs plus one cup of liquid such as coconut milk. (You can also add cooked, puréed, or mashed fruit or vegetables to increase the moisture.) Or you can mix it with all-purpose flour.

Try it in: Breads, cakes, muffins, cookies, pancakes

Whole-grain oat flour

Whole-grain oat flour is made from pure oats, so it has all of their outstanding qualities: lots of fiber (5 grams per ½ cup) and protein. It's also another great option for those with a gluten allergy or sensitivity. The oats add a nutty flavor and a dense or chewy texture to whatever you incorporate them into.

How to use it: Since oat flour doesn't contain gluten, you will need to adjust your ingredients to make your baked items light and fluffy. In baked goods that need to rise, it needs to be combined; replace up to 20 percent of the flour in baking recipes.

Try it in: Bran muffins, zucchini bread, carrot cake, oatmeal raisin cookies

Spelt flour

Spelt is an organic whole grain—it's tricky in the sense that it's nonwheat but it's still not gluten free. (They're in the same grain family but are different species with different properties. That's important to remember if you are avoiding gluten.) It, too, has a nutty flavor.

How to use it: Try it in any recipe that you'd use whole-wheat flour for, but swapping in less—up to 20 percent of the called-for flour for spelt flour.

Try it in: Breads, pizza crust, tortillas, cakes, pasta noodles

Even more variations

Grinding up foods into flour doesn't stop with the above options. If you're looking to experiment with tastes and textures, you can use amaranth, arrowroot, barley, buckwheat, chickpeas, millet, potatoes, sweet potatoes, quinoa, rice, rye, soy, tapioca, and teff. These flours may be harder to find—you'll have the best luck at specialty grocery stores or online—but are more nutritionally valuable than standard all-purpose flour.

THE INGREDIENT: Milk

Cow's milk is famously loaded with protein, calcium, and vitamin D. It's such a stellar source of calcium, in fact, that it's practically synonymous with strong, healthy bones. But there's one small problem: it's deceptively high in sugar. Regardless of whether it's whole milk or low-fat milk, 1 cup contains about 12 grams of sugar. Yes, it's natural sugar—in milk, it's called lactose—but too much sugar, regardless of where it comes from, can have some seriously negative effects. And when it's in a seemingly healthy food like milk, it still adds up quickly if you're drinking a glass with every meal. The bottom line here is that you don't need to stop drinking dairy milk, but you should be aware of what it can and cannot do for your body. Plus, there are lots of nondairy options out there that are packed with similar nutrients but lower in sugar or even sugar free.

The Substitutions:

Try these in: Smoothies, cereal, salad dressings, pudding, soups, coffee, Mashed Cauliflower (see page 96), or by the glass

Unsweetened almond milk

Almond milk has been enjoying a surge in popularity, and it's well deserved. It has about half the calories of cow's milk and zero cholesterol. That's precisely why I included it as one of my all-star ingredients—flip to page 56 for the rundown on its other nutritional perks.

How to use it: Stick with unsweetened original and unsweetened vanilla options, which contain zero natural or added sugar.

Unsweetened cashew milk

Cashew milk is a lot like almond milk: it contains little to no saturated fat and cholesterol; it's also smooth, creamy, flavorful, and dairy free. The major difference in this nut milk is that it's, well, made from the milk of cashews.

How to use it: Again, like with almond milk, stick with the unsweetened version, which contains little to no sugar.

Coconut milk

You know a milk alternative has made a splash when Starbucks begins to offer it, as is the case with coconut milk. The good: coconut milk is very low in cholesterol and sodium, in addition to being dairy free, better for your heart than cow's milk, and full of that distinctive nutty flavor. The bad: traditional coconut milk is extremely high in saturated fat—it contains more than even whole milk, with one cup serving up two and a half times the suggested daily value. Yikes.

How to use it: Buy the light version, which can slash its saturated fat and calories in half or more. If you're intent on the traditional version, use it sparingly—that means an occasional splash in your coffee. I find it to be very sweet, so you won't need much more than that.

Soy milk

Soy milk is not for everyone, and not just because of its unique taste. For every pro, there seems to be a corresponding con. It's cholesterol free and high in good fats, so it's great for your heart health—but you need to consume a lot of soy to see the effects. However, consuming *too* much soy has been associated with the speeding up of brain cell aging and messing with your thyroid.

How to use it: Soy allergies and sensitivities are extremely common, so listen to your body. Opt for soy if you truly enjoy the taste, and consume it in moderation.

Rice milk

Another option for those avoiding dairy is rice milk, which is made from ground rice. It's low in fat (yay!) but also low in protein (boo).

How to use it: If rice milk becomes your go-to milk alternative, either up your protein intake elsewhere in your diet or find a brand that comes fortified with calcium and/or vitamin D so you're getting some nutrients.

THE INGREDIENT: Butter or Margarine

Neither butter nor margarine is ideal in your diet, and it mostly comes down to the specific fats that they contain. Just one tablespoon of butter has 11 grams of fat, and 7 grams of that is saturated fat—that's more than a third of the recommended daily amount. (Reminder: saturated fats have long been linked to poor heart health/high cholesterol.) One tablespoon of margarine, meanwhile, has less saturated fat than butter—2.2 grams—but also 2.1 grams of trans fat. Trans fat is the worst kind of dietary fat, even in small amounts, because of the havoc it wreaks on your cholesterol in addition to being linked to heart disease and diabetes. But it's also worth noting that in recent years, butter's public image has been on the upswing and scientists are reexamining its true detriment to your health. In the meantime, play around with these alternatives in your recipes by mixing them with butter or replacing it all.

The Substitutions:

Coconut oil

Coconut oil isn't overwhelmingly healthier than butter, since it has more saturated and calories. But it's lower in cholesterol and has that nutty flavor—so you may be inclined to use less.

How to use it: In baked goods, sub in coconut oil for butter in a 1:1 ratio.

Try it in: Muffins, cakes, banana or pumpkin bread, waffles

Unsweetened applesauce

You've probably heard of this trick before: replace the butter or oil in baking recipes with unsweetened applesauce. In with the fruit, out with the fat. It'll provide the same consistency and a slight sweetness. Note the increased natural sugar.

How to use it: If you don't think you'll mind a slightly spongier end product, swap in unsweetened applesauce in a 1:1 ratio (a half cup of applesauce for a half cup of butter). You can also use it to replace eggs.

Try it in: Pancakes, fruity or spiced breads, muffins, brownies, oatmeal cookies

Mashed or puréed avocado

Okay, now we're starting to get outside the box. Avocados—one of my all-star foods (see page 59 for even more additional uses)— have a similar texture to butter as well as more "good" fat. They will add moisture and produce less crumbliness.

How to use it: After being mashed, avocados technically work in a 1:1 ratio in recipes that call for butter. But they won't react quite the same with dry ingredients; to fix this, you can either increase the amount of wet ingredients or use a half-butter, half-avocado combo.

Try it in: Banana or zucchini breads, muffins, any baked good with chocolate

Buttery spread

It's not butter—it's a vague term called *buttery spread* and designed to mimic butter's color, consistency, and taste. And it's not the healthiest alternative, considering it's categorized as a processed food (just check out that lengthy ingredients list!) and still contains sodium. But there's one notable perk: Earth Balance, Smart Balance, and Olivio offer options that can lower cholesterol while containing about only 2 or less grams of saturated fat and little to no trans fat.

How to use it: Again, buttery spreads certainly aren't considered a superfood—they're just as fatty as real-deal butter. Buttery spreads are ideal if you're concerned about your cholesterol. Always read the nutrition label, looking for options with little to no trans fat, and use it in moderation.

Try it in: Popcorn, Zucchini Noodles (see page 93), Whole-Wheat Crepes (see page 76)

THE INGREDIENT: Sugar

I've gotten to the point where I have zero tolerance for added sugar: you won't find a grain of table sugar in my house because I haven't bought it in years. It doesn't provide any nutrients to the food it's added to, so I've simply eliminated it from the equation. That may sound drastic (or ridiculous), but thanks to a few natural sweeteners that also supply nutrients, my life is still pretty sweet.

Try these sweeteners in: Nuts, muffins, pancakes, coffee

The Substitutions:

Maple syrup

Pure maple syrup is three times as sweet as table sugar and has half the calories. It's a good source of manganese and zinc and also contains calcium, iron, and potassium.

How to use it: Look for 100 percent pure maple syrup—it should be the only ingredient in the bottle. (Skip the imitation stuff, which usually contains corn syrup.) In baking, the conversion rate is about ⅔ cup to ¾ cup of maple syrup per cup of refined sugar.

Agave nectar

Agave nectar has 20 calories per teaspoon, 5 more than granulated sugar, but because it's sweeter, you can use less of it. It also contains more fructose, meaning it's less likely to make your blood sugar surge.

How to use it: A generally accepted rule is to use one-third less agave nectar than you would white sugar and then reduce other liquids in the recipe by one-fourth.

Honey

Honey contains a tiny amount of vitamins like niacin, riboflavin, and thiamin. It can also soothe a sore throat—when was the last time a sugar cube did that?

How to use it: Some people replace sugar with just as much honey, but try to reduce it to ⅔ or ¾ of the called-for amount since it's on par with sugar in terms of calories.

Stevia or Truvia

Stevia is a plant in the chrysanthemum family that's native to Paraguay; Truvia is a brand of sweetener products made from stevia leaves. Stevia in the raw and Truvia are both zero-calorie sweeteners. Neither is FDA-approved, but stevia has the next best thing: the FDA's "generally recognized as safe" certification.

How to use it: Truvia's extreme sweetness allows it to be used super sparingly: one-quarter of the amount of sugar or less.

PART 3

GETTING LEAN

CHAPTER 9

The 4-Minute Workout

Early in my career, I often trained my clients with lots of clas- sic circuit moves. They were fun and effective, and I was constantly looking for ways to put a twist on them. Then, sometime around 2012, I read an article about an incredibly ef- fective method of exercise called tabata: a four-minute workout that's broken into eight rounds of intense exercise for twenty sec- onds, then ten seconds of rest. Intrigued, I tried it myself. I was hooked immediately.

Now's a great time to stop and explain that what I call ta- bata workouts are actually variations on the original tabata method, which was studied by (and named after) a sport and health-science researcher named Izumi Tabata. He was also a training coach with the Japanese Olympic speed-skating team, whose head coach had developed a specific high-intensity inter- val training regimen for his athletes. Dr. Tabata was asked to analyze this regimen's effectiveness, leading to a landmark study that was published in the journal *Medicine and Science in Sports and Exercise* in 1996. The study itself is long and dense, so I've lifted only the most important info from it here. Bear with me, because its findings are why my tabata workouts are so effective.

Here's what happened in the study: Dr. Tabata, who trans- formed from speed-skating coach to researcher, gathered a group of male college students and conducted two experiments over six weeks. In the first experiment, the participants rode a station- ary bike at moderate intensity for one hour, five days a week. In the second experiment, the participants pedaled on a stationary bike as hard as they could for twenty seconds—we're talking all-out exertion, like they were about to pass out—then rested for ten seconds; they did this a total of eight times, or as many times as they could. (Dr. Tabata reportedly told them, "If you feel okay afterward, you've not done it properly.") Group two did this four-minute workout four times a week.

After six weeks, Dr. Tabata and his research team analyzed two factors:

- the participants' anaerobic capacity, which is how long you can perform an exercise with maximum exertion
- the participants' VO_2 max, which is the highest amount of oxygen your body can consume and use for energy

The results were stunning: the young men who biked at a consistent moderate rate improved their VO_2 max by 10 percent, and their steady cycling regimen had no effect on their anaerobic capacity. But the young men who'd worked out in four-minute bursts? They improved their VO_2 max significantly—and upped their anaerobic capacity by 28 percent. There are lots of variables to consider here (like that all students involved in the study were already physically fit), but basically the study showed that four minutes of high-intensity cycling was significantly more effective than an entire hour of moderate cycling.

So back to my stumbling upon this totally innovative concept and my brain jumping into action. The original tabata protocol used a stationary bike, but why stop at cardio? I decided to take the idea of the four-minute workout and apply it to the regular exercise moves I'd been doing myself and with my clients for years.

I downloaded a tabata timer app on my phone and went out in my front yard, trying out all sorts of moves in twenty-second bursts, followed by ten seconds of rest. Squats, and all their variations? Yup, those worked. Sit-ups, and all their variations? Those too! Hammer curls? Yes—tabata-style workouts, I discovered, are especially awesome with weights.

I became obsessed with tabatas, combining my "old" exercises and this "new" style. I played around with different moves and sequences every day for about a week—seeing which exercises worked best in the tabata format and monitoring how I felt afterward. (I ended up doing ten to fifteen tabatas each day because I was so excited to test them out. I don't recommend this—I was so sore afterward!) I loved how much stronger my cardiovascular system felt and, just as importantly, that there's an endless number of tabata combinations to create.

Then I started rolling out my version of the tabata method with my clients. I did this slowly and carefully. Could they do tabata-style workouts? Would it be effective? Would they actually like it? I soon learned the answers: yes, yes, and yes.

Here are four reasons my clients and I love incorporating tabata into workouts:

1. It's like a game.

Personally, I consider any kind of workout "fun"—but I know not everyone thinks that way. Many of my clients tell me that they love how tabatas can turn a run-of-the-mill workout into a fast-paced game. It's you against the timer.

Even the tabata app is on board with this idea: it ticks down the seconds you have left of each exercise, and when it's time to start going again, it dings like it's kicking off a boxing match. (Learn more about using the tabata timer on page 123.) You don't want to lose, right?

2. You can do *anything* for twenty seconds.

What's your least favorite workout move? You know, the one that makes you groan just thinking about it. Maybe you struggle with push-ups or you think planks are impossibly boring. Now, what if you only had to do that dreaded move for twenty seconds at a time, and then you got a quick break? Incorporating tabata is a game-changer, mentally as well as physically: You're not doing 100 push-ups. You're not holding a plank for two minutes. You're just doing it for twenty seconds, and then you have ten seconds to rest your body. It's become a mantra for many of my clients: "You can do anything for twenty seconds."

3. It's structured.

Too many times, I've seen people working out with very clearly no plan in mind. A few bicep curls, a few squats, and a whole lot of facial expressions that seem to say "Now what?" Talk about inefficient! It's the opposite with tabatas. Once you pick a tabata to do, there is no question of what move is coming in the next round. Bonus: the constant movement also makes the time fly by.

4. You can mix and match your favorite moves.

In one sense, tabatas are structured; in another, they're really flexible. As I've mentioned, you can apply the tabata style to hundreds of basic workout moves. In Chapter 12, I lay out my favorites in three categories: Beginner, Intermediate, and Advanced. You'll find a good mix of exercise types and target areas; I've also included several cardio tabatas that you can do on a treadmill or stationary bike to mix up your routine.

But I couldn't include every move I use—there are simply too many to fit into a book. On page 194, I walk you through five of the easiest ways to modify any tabata. In addition, you can apply the tabata format to cardio training, plyometrics, and body-weight moves that I didn't include here. All you need is twenty seconds of intensity, followed by ten seconds of rest. That means you'll have to try *really* hard to get bored with these super-powered exercises.

CHAPTER 10

The Equipment You'll Need

When I was starting out in my personal training career, I worked out of a studio and had clients come to me. Then I started my own company—and ever since, I either go to my clients' houses to train or meet them at a park or other outdoor area. Everything we could possibly need for a workout fits in the back of my car, and every workout can be done in the space of a small room.

Many of the 4 × 4 tabatas do not require any equipment other than a timer, but some do. Here is the equipment you'll need for all three levels of tabatas. As you'll see, there's a lot of flexibility here; you don't need to go out and buy the latest or most expensive models from specialty stores. All of these items can be found at sporting goods stores and major retailers like Walmart and Target.

Now, I'm definitely not opposed to gyms. I belong to a local gym and go whenever I have downtime between training sessions or if the weather is nasty. I'm also a huge fan of cardio tabatas, which can be done on a treadmill or stationary bike (find those on page 192). But it's important to know that if you don't want to pay the membership costs or there are no suitable facilities near you, you don't need to belong to a gym.

Tabata Timer

This is the most important piece of equipment you'll need for tabatas— it's the only thing you'll *really* need for every single workout. There are quite a few options to download for both iOS and Android, including Interval Timer, Tabata Stopwatch, and Bit Timer. I use the Interval Timer app for iOS because it's straightforward and free.

Yoga Mat

No need to be picky with your mat—any thickness, any material works. Just remember to give it a quick wipe-down after every few uses, at a minimum.

Dumbbells

You'll want to get three sets of these versatile weights: light, medium, heavy. You'll use them for moves like arm curls and shoulder presses, and you can add weights to certain nonweighted moves to make them harder (see page 195 for more on this kind of tabata modification). The exact weights needed will vary from person to person; they should fall between 3 and 25 pounds. My recommendation: start with a set of 3-pounders as your light weights, a set of 5-pounders as your medium weights, and a set of 8-pounders as your heavy weights. Once the 3s become easy to use as your light weights, replace them with 5s and bump up the rest accordingly.

Jump Rope

Just as with the yoga mat, any brand of jump rope will do. Pick one that you will be excited to use—look for your favorite color or handles that are super comfortable to grip.

The rope should just skim the ground as you swing it. If it's too long, you can shorten it by knotting the side of the rope one or two times. And if it breaks, consider it a fitness victory. I break jump ropes all the time from using them so much!

Resistance Bands

There are different levels of resistance bands, anywhere from extra light to extra heavy. I recommend having light, medium, and heavy. You can use these in place of dumbbells for exercises like curls, bent-over rows, and lateral raises.

Resistance bands have one major advantage over dumbbells: they're extremely portable. Throw one in your suitcase the next time you're traveling so you can work out on the road.

Foam Roller

While it's not used in any of the actual tabatas, the foam roller is a crucial part of your postworkout stretch. Most rollers are 6 inches in diameter, and they can range from 12 inches to 36 inches long. The more dense the roller, the more effective it will be in stretching you out. I further my case for the foam roller—and give several ways to use it—on page 130.

For me, this tool is essential after a soccer game or extra-hard workout. Foam rolling is one of the only things that truly relaxes the tightness through my hips. My clients, too, have fallen in love with these stretches—I even bought one of my clients a foam roller for Christmas.

CHAPTER 11

Before and After Every Workout

There's more to every workout than just the actual workout. But don't be alarmed: these "extras" are easy to do and should make your body feel *good*. Bookending each workout with a warm-up and a cooldown keeps your body healthy enough to maintain a regular exercise regimen in addition to providing a host of other benefits. Just a few simple moves pre- and postworkout will allow you to get the most out of all the hard work you put in.

Warming Up

Before doing a workout of any kind, it's crucial to warm up your body. A proper warm-up should take five to ten minutes and will ease you into what lies ahead, both physically and psychologically. Dedicate this time to lubing up your muscles and your brain, politely letting them know they are about to be put to work.

Just five to ten minutes of moderate movement provides head-to-toe benefits. Your warm-up will increase your blood flow, which in turn lessens stiffness in your muscles. You'll notice an improved range of motion, too, especially in joints like your hips. A good warm-up also literally warms you up—as in your muscles, your body temperature, and your blood temperature—

which can lead to better muscle elasticity, reduced risk of strains and pulls, and a boost in overall performance. Lastly, but just as important, consider your warm-up a mental preparation for your workout. Clear your mind so you can focus fully on the upcoming exercises—some people call this "getting in the zone."

Just as there are different levels of workouts (including tabatas), there are different levels of warm-ups. The following moves are simple but perfect for a proper warm-up:

· Walking
· Lightly jogging
· Jumping jacks
· High-knee running in place
· Skipping
· Jumping rope

The above warm-up moves progress in difficulty, so if you're new to working out, start by walking for about five minutes. As your fitness level increases, you can make your warm-up more challenging by incorporating a couple of minutes of light jogging. Kick it up even more by combining other moves: alternate jumping jacks and skipping or jumping rope and running with high knees. Just make sure to put in the time before each and every workout—your body will (silently) thank you.

Cooling Down

After every workout, a cooldown period is as important as the warm-up that kicked things off. Both mentally and physically, it informs your body that it has completed what you have asked of it. Mission accomplished! Done properly, a postworkout stretch provides some of the same benefits as your warm-up: it improves your flexibility, increases blood flow, boosts the range of motion in your joints, and reduces your risk of injury. A cooldown also keeps your muscles limber since it's likely that they are tight from being worked.

Get in the habit of stretching your major muscle groups—quads, hamstrings, glutes, back, chest, shoulders, neck—plus any other groups or areas you just worked. Always stretch immediately after your workout, while your muscles are still loose and warm.

Here are my go-to postworkout stretches. Do each one for twenty to thirty seconds.

Quads

Stand on your right leg, grab your left ankle with your left hand, and pull your left heel to your left glute. You should feel the stretch in the front of your left leg. Repeat on the opposite side. If you need balance, use the back of a chair or a pole.

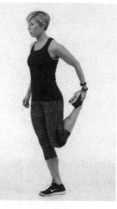

You can also do this stretch lying on your side.

Hamstrings

Lie on your back and lift and straighten your left leg above your hips. Hold your left calf and press your left heel toward the ceiling as you pull your leg back toward your chest; keep both legs straight for the whole stretch. Switch legs.

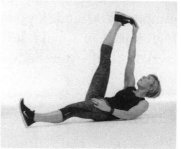

If you can't reach your leg to pull it back, loop a towel or exercise band around the bottom of your foot and then pull slowly.

Glutes

Lying on your back, cross your left leg over your bent right knee. Grab

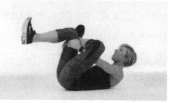

your right leg with both hands and pull back slowly toward your chest, feeling the stretch in your butt and hip.

To feel a deeper stretch, gently push your left knee out.

Back

Go on all fours and arch your back upward, like an angry cat, and hold. Then arch your back under, pushing your lower back toward the ground, and hold. Repeat as needed.

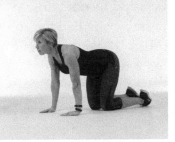

Most of my clients automatically do this move after planks and back workouts like skydivers (see page 147 for skydiver instructions).

Chest

Stand up straight, with your fingers laced behind your back. Now straighten your arms and push your chest forward.

If you can't reach your hands behind your back, place your right palm on a door frame, straighten your right arm, and twist your body away from the frame. Switch sides.

Triceps

Stand up straight and raise your right arm, then bend it so that your right hand goes past your head, and reach down your spine. Use your left hand to further push your right elbow down. Switch arms.

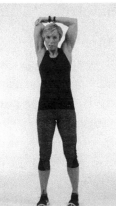

Stretching with a Foam Roller

Foam rollers are really an unsung hero in the fitness world. They're inexpensive (often less than $20), you can use them on virtually any body part, and their unique combination of softness and firmness allows you to stretch out specific areas of soreness. I wish I had the ability to give everyone in the world a foam roller. While I work out the logistics of that goal, master these foam-rolling tips:

- **Speeding through the motions is wasting the roll.** Use slow, purposeful motions. Draw . . . them . . . out . . . like . . . this.
- **Focus on the areas that are most painful.** Hold on each sore area for a good ten seconds before moving on to another spot. You can even hold on an area until it softens and becomes less painful or relaxing.
- **Your first few foam-rolling sessions should be short.** Start by rolling for just a few minutes, and slowly increase the length of the session over the next few weeks. Eventually, you can roll for five to fifteen minutes, based on your soreness.

Try these stretches at least three times per week, whenever you're sore:

Hamstring/Glutes

Sit on the roller with the soft part of your butt on top of the roller. Roll back and forth slowly, moving from your butt through your hamstrings to the back of your knees, and repeat. Throughout, stop and hold the pressure on your sore spots.

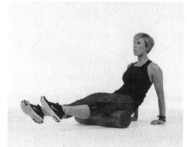

Quads

Lie on top of the roller, with your quads over the foam and using your hands as support. Roll slowly along the muscle.

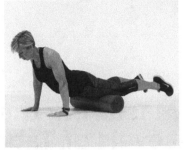

IT Band

Place your left hip on the roller
and slowly roll down to the side of your left knee. As you roll, stop and hold at tender areas. Repeat on your right side.

Your IT band runs along the side of each leg, all the way up through your hip.

Upper/Lower Back

Lie with the roller underneath you, positioned under your shoulder blades or lower lumbar. Support your head with your hands and roll back and forth, planting your feet for support and movement.

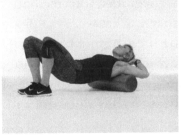
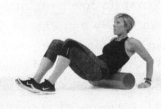

CHAPTER 12

Mastering the Three Levels of Tabatas

Any time you try a new fitness regimen, even if you consider yourself to be pretty fit, don't expect to master it immediately. With tabatas, you'll be doing twenty-second bursts of intense exercise, and it may take a few weeks to become accustomed to how they affect your body. Also, you'll be incorporating a timer into your workouts, which may be tricky at first. Finally—and this goes for any kind of workout—if you take on too much too soon, you have a higher chance of not seeing it through (and possibly getting injured doing it). So start slowly and be patient!

In this chapter, I'll show you thirty of my favorite tabatas. I've broken them down into three levels: Beginner, Intermediate, and Advanced. No matter your fitness level, start with the Beginner Tabatas so you can get used to the four-minute pattern; if you find these to be easy right away, move up to Intermediate Tabatas without waiting a week. You'll know you're ready to move on to the next level once you continue through the full tabata without feeling challenged.

As always, you need to listen to your body. Some people don't push themselves hard enough and some people push themselves too hard—the trick is finding the sweet spot between the two. It's an awareness that you'll develop as you become leaner and cleaner. I call it a healthy addiction: as you start to see changes in your body, you'll want to keep pushing and challenging yourself. Then it becomes key to create your own tabatas by combining your favorite moves or tweaking the ones I show you (learn more about that on page 194).

Incorporating Tabatas into the 4 × 4 Diet

These thirty tabatas are the tools you'll use for the lean part of the 4 × 4 Diet—lasting just four minutes each, they are the second "4." Here's how you'll use them: each week, aim to do three or four workouts. Each of those workouts should consist of four to six tabatas, and you'll start by choosing from the ones I show you below. (One tabata is like a mini workout in which you perform several moves.) Each of these thirty tabatas consists of eight thirty-second rounds—that's twenty seconds of intense exercise, then ten seconds of rest—lasting four minutes total. It all comes back to the number 4.

**That's a lot of numbers.
So before we move on, let's go over that again:**

- One tabata lasts eight rounds, and each is twenty seconds of exercise, ten seconds of rest.
- String together four to six of these eight-round tabatas for a complete workout. (That's only sixteen to twenty-four minutes of exercise total!)
- Complete a tabata workout three or four times per week.

Got it?

Now, many of these tabatas—and all of the Beginner Tabatas—consist of four different moves for eight rounds. So in these tabatas, you'll do each move twice: Rounds 1 and 5 are the same move; rounds 2 and 6 are the same move; rounds 3 and 7 are the same move; and rounds 4 and 8 are the same move. A harder version is doing two moves, four times each, and you'll find a few of these among the Intermediate Tabatas. The hardest option is doing the same move for all eight rounds. When you're ready for Advanced Tabatas, you'll tackle some of these.

If This Sounds Complicated, Don't Worry

You know how when you try to explain something that's incredibly simple, it can come out sounding incredibly complicated?

That's how I feel about tabatas. But they can be easily learned—my clients will attest to that—and I'm going to walk you through the process. Grab your timer and let's do a test run.

Beginner Tabatas

Welcome to Beginner Tabatas! During the first week of the 4 × 4 Diet, unless you're already extremely active, you'll be doing moves only from this level. Here, I give you ten Beginner Tabatas, each consisting of four consecutive moves that you'll repeat, for a total of eight rounds. Test out each tabata to see which ones you like most and can do best—it's okay to repeat tabatas as you master them.

Stick with these Beginner Tabatas for at least a week, as you get the hang of the tabata method and ramp up your activity level. (Don't forget, you're still working toward taking 10,000 steps per day.) In weeks 2 and 3, you'll be working in Intermediate Tabatas—those will be a bit harder and more intense.

Here's why I want you to do only Beginner Tabatas for the first week or two:

There's minimal vertical movement. You won't find yourself going up and down—too much, at least—with these moves. If you're up you stay up, and if you're down you stay down.

The muscle groups are spread out. If you work the same group of muscles back-to-back, they're more difficult. So we'll get to those later!

The intensity is limited. Moves that involve jumping (like jumping jacks in Beginner Tabata #2) increase your heart rate. But since you want to start out slow, these tabatas avoid consecutive moves that boost your heart rate.

They consist of four different moves. Every tabata has eight rounds. When you're doing one move eight times in a row, it's a lot harder on whatever part of your body you are working. Mixing them up—in this case, four moves each done twice—will reduce the strain.

Many moves are modified from a harder version. For example, the push-ups in Beginner Tabatas #1 and #6 are done on your knees; this way, you don't have to lift your entire body weight—just your upper body.

BEGINNER TABATA #1

Round 1: Knee Push-ups
Works your chest, core, and triceps

Go on your knees with your hands just wider than your shoulders, feet up, core engaged, and back flat. Perform a push-up. Return to the starting position.

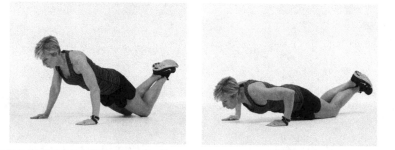

If putting weight on your knees is painful, try using a wall or a step to perform a beginner-level push-up. However you end up performing these push-ups, make sure you challenge yourself.

Round 2: Floor Dips
Works your triceps

Sit on your butt, bend your knees, and go on your heels. Place your hands next to your glutes with your fingers pointing toward your feet. Raise your hips up and bend your elbows, shooting them straight back, then push back up.

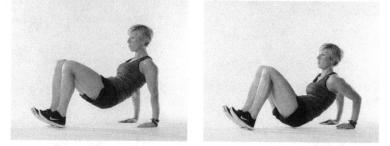

Don't just lower your butt to the floor—actually bend your elbows! And if the floor is too uncomfortable, use a step or chair instead.

Round 3: Right Leg Bridge Pulses
Works your hamstrings, glutes, and core

Lie on your back, bend your left leg, and go on your left heel. Bring your right leg and hips straight up in the air and push up and down, never letting your hips hit the ground.

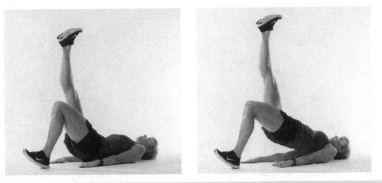

If you can't raise one leg, perform these with both feet down for two consecutive rounds.

Round 4: Left Leg Bridge Pulses
Works your hamstrings, glutes, and core

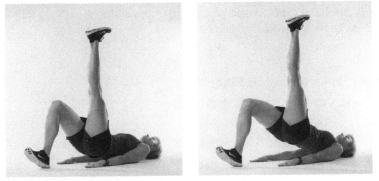

Lie on your back, bend your right leg, and go on your right heel. Bring your left leg and hips straight up in the air and push up and down, never letting your hips hit the ground.

Repeat rounds 1–4.

BEGINNER TABATA #2
All cardio

Round 1: Jumping Jacks

Stand upright with your feet together and your arms by your sides. Jump and land with your feet shoulder width apart, simultaneously raising your arms overhead. Jump back to starting position.

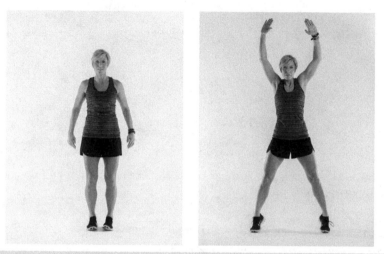

If you feel significant pain while jumping, try doing the same arm movements but either tapping one foot out to the side at a time or marching in place (with high knees, if possible).

Round 2: Running in Place

Hop from foot to foot, driving your arms forward.

If the pounding motion is severely uncomfortable, try stepping rapidly in place.

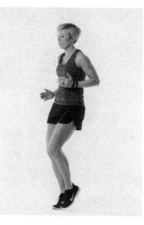

Round 3: Mountain Climbers

Get into plank position with your back flat and hands straight below your shoulders. Keeping your core tight, bring one knee toward your chest, then take it back; switch legs. You should feel like you're running in place in prone position.

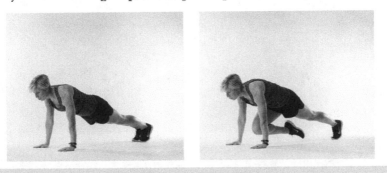

Go as slowly as you need to while starting out.

Round 4: Cross Jumping Jacks

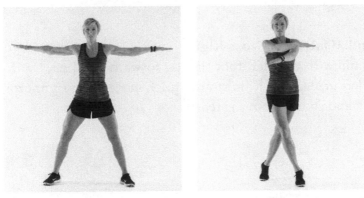

As you jump, your arms and legs will cross in front of you. Keep your arms at shoulder level throughout the exercise.

Repeat rounds 1–4.

BEGINNER TABATA #3
All cardio

Round 1: Straight Punches

Stand square and punch straight out at shoulder level with your right hand, then your left hand. Keep your knees soft and abs tight.

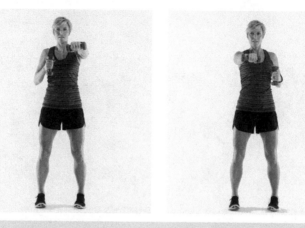

To get the most out of this move, you need to punch quickly and keep your core super engaged.

Round 2: Jab Left, Cross Right

Stand with your left foot slightly forward and knees soft. Jab your left arm out in a short and quick movement; right cross is longer and comes from the rear.

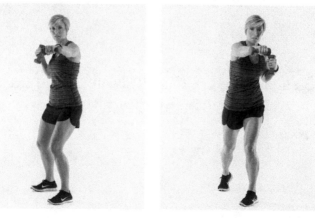

Round 3: Jab Right, Cross Left

Stand with your right foot slightly forward and knees soft. Jab your right arm out in a short and quick movement; left cross is longer and comes from the rear.

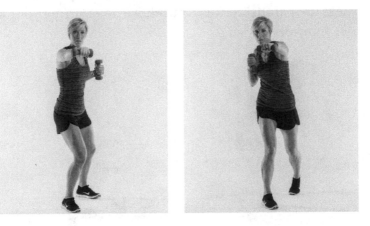

Round 4: Hook Punches

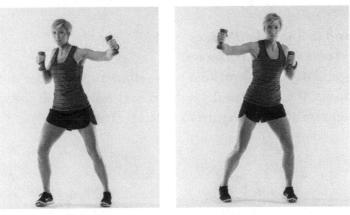

Stand square, knees soft, arms raised to your sides. Bend your right elbow forward 90 degrees and swing that arm forward in a horizontal arc. Repeat with your left arm.

Repeat rounds 1–4.

Add 3- to 5-pound weights once you've mastered these air punches.

BEGINNER TABATA #4

Round 1: Squats
Works your quads, glutes, and hamstrings

Stand with your legs shoulder width apart, pelvis rotated back, weight on your heels, and head and chest up. Sit down until your legs are parallel to the ground, without letting your knees go past your toes.

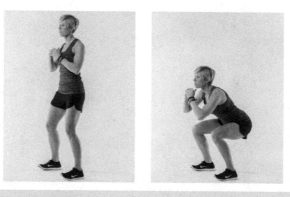

For any kind of squat or lunge move, hold onto a door frame or railing if you need extra balance.

Round 2: Shoulder Presses
Works your shoulders and triceps

Stand with your arms out wide, elbows at shoulder level, and holding a 5- to 15-pound weight in each hand. Push the weights straight up and then return to shoulder level.

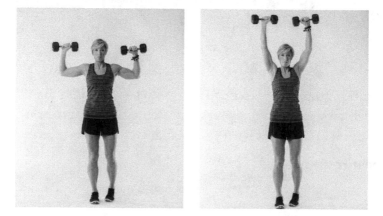

Round 3: Sumo Squats

Works your inner thighs, quads, and glutes

Stand with your legs out wide, toes at a 45-degree angle. Drop your butt until your legs are parallel to the ground, keeping your weight on your heels. Return to starting position.

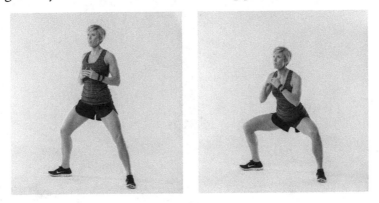

Round 4: Bicep Curls

Works your biceps

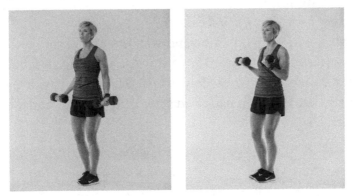

Grab a pair of 5- to 15-pound weights, turn your palms up, and curl the weights upward, keeping your elbows glued to your sides.

Repeat rounds 1–4.

BEGINNER TABATA #5

Round 1: Reverse Lunge Switch
Works your quads, hamstrings, and glutes

Stand on your left leg and take your right leg back into a lunge. Drop your right knee straight to the ground. Pushing off your front heel, return to starting position. Switch legs.

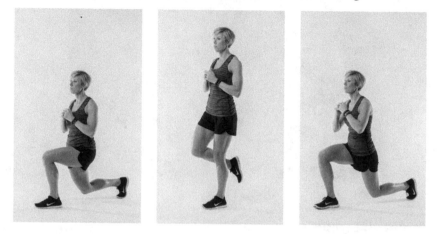

Round 2: Bent-Over Rows
Works your back, biceps, and shoulders

Grab a pair of 5- to 15-pound weights and stand with your knees softened. Fall forward at your waist, keeping your back flat and extending your arms downward. Then bend your elbows, shooting them straight back and squeezing your shoulder blades together.

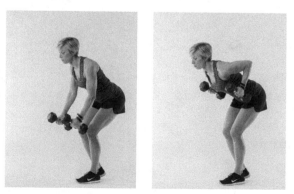

Round 3: High-Knee Elbow Taps
Cardio

Stand straight, hands behind your head. Bring your right knee high toward your left elbow. Repeat with left leg.

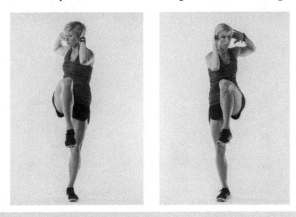

Keep your chest tall—do not bend down to your knee.

Round 4: Lateral Raises
Works your shoulders

Grab a pair of 5- to 15-pound weights, bend your elbows slightly, and keep your knees soft. Raise your arms straight out to the sides, up to shoulder level, elbows still soft. Lower to starting position.

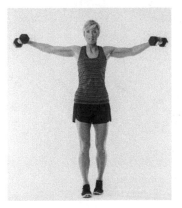

Repeat rounds 1–4.

BEGINNER TABATA #6

Round 1: High Plank
Works your core

Start in a plank position with your hands shoulder width apart. Engage your abs, squeeze your butt and quads, and do not let your butt elevate into the air or dip toward the floor. Hold.

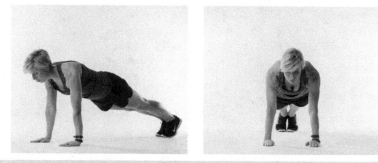

Your hands should be closer together than they would be for a push-up.

Round 2: Knee Push-ups
Works your chest, triceps, and core

Go on your knees with hands just wider than your shoulders, feet up, core engaged, and back flat. Perform a push-up. Return to starting position, keeping your hips tucked throughout the maneuver.

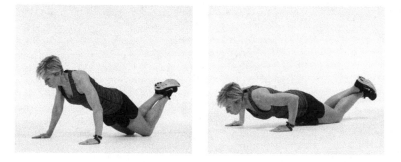

Round 3: Skydivers
Works your lower back, glutes, and hamstrings

Lie on your stomach and stretch your arms behind you, as if you're diving headfirst out of a plane. Arch your chest and lift your head, shoulders, and chest while also lifting your feet as high as you can. Dip your chin in to relax your neck.

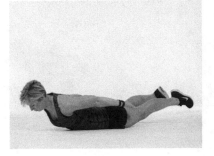

Round 4: Tippy-Toe Bridges
Works your calves, core, hamstrings, and glutes

Lie on your back, arms at your sides, knees bent. Stand on your tippy-toes and push your hips up. Thrust your hips up and down, keeping your heels raised and never letting your butt hit the ground.

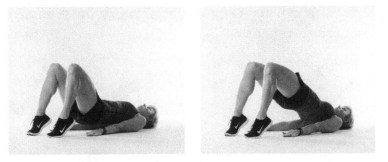

Repeat rounds 1–4.

BEGINNER TABATA #7

Round 1: Hammer Curls
Works your biceps

Grab a pair of 5- to 10-pound weights and grip them with your thumbs facing up. Keeping your elbows glued to your sides, curl your arms upward with your thumbs facing up.

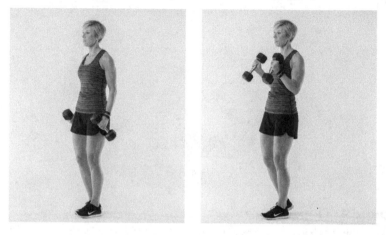

Round 2: Tricep Kickbacks
Works your triceps

Grab a pair of 5- to 10-pound weights and fall forward at your waist, with your back flat and elbows bent 90 degrees at your sides. Extend both arms straight back, squeezing your triceps. Return to starting position.

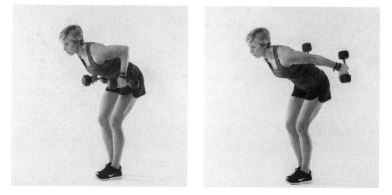

Round 3: Small Arm Rotations

Works your shoulders

Extend your arms straight out to your sides at shoulder level and make tiny forward-motion circles in the air. Keep your arms locked.

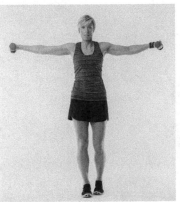

Add up to a 5-pound weight once you get the hang of this move.

Round 4: V Front Raise

Works your shoulders

Start with your arms at your sides, holding a pair of 3- to 10-pound weights. Raise them in front of you up to shoulder level, creating a V in the air. Reverse in a controlled manner to return to starting position.

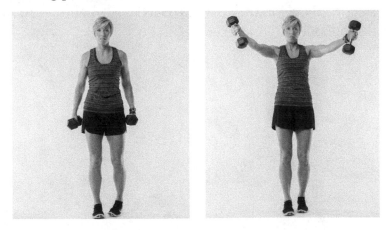

Repeat rounds 1–4.

BEGINNER TABATA #8

Round 1: Pretend Jump Rope
Cardio

Swing your arms and jump over the "rope," keeping your elbows glued to your sides.

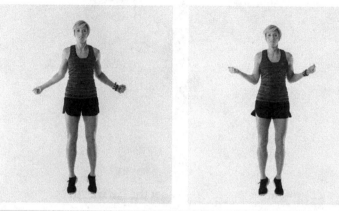

If this move is too intense, combine rapid high stepping in place with arm rotations.

Round 2: Side Shuffle
Cardio + works your quads

Assume a squat position, rotate your hips back, and shuffle five steps to the right, then five to the left. It's important to stay low throughout the entire exercise.

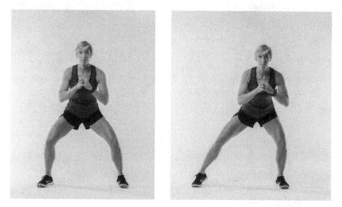

Round 3: Windmills

Cardio

Reach your right arm toward your left foot while your left arm stays straight and extends upward. Keep your arms rigid and stand up as you raise them wide to shoulder level. Switch sides.

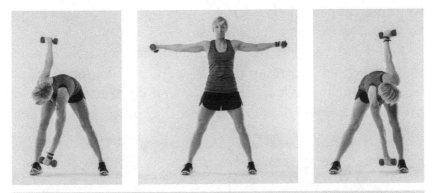

Once you've mastered this form of old-school calisthenics, add up to 10-pound weights.

Round 4: Squat Holds

Cardio + works your quads

Sit back on your heels, dropping down until your upper legs are parallel to the floor. Hold for the entire twenty seconds; it should burn! Try to stay low the entire time; if you're not at that level, come up slightly and hold there—don't stand all the way.

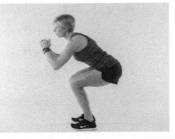

If you're near a wall, put your back flat against it and perform the move.

Repeat rounds 1–4.

BEGINNER TABATA #9

You'll need a bench for all four of these moves. A step, chair, or ottoman will work too!

Round 1: Step Up (Left Leg)
Works your quads, hamstrings, and glutes

Stand with your left foot on the bench and your right foot on the floor behind it. Lift your right knee up, balancing on your left leg, then touch it back on the ground and immediately shoot it back up. Keep your left foot on the bench throughout.

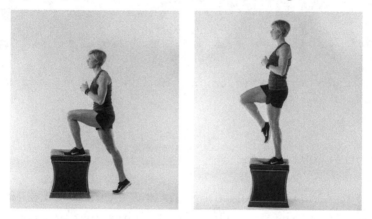

Round 2: Bench Dips
Works your triceps

Sit on the bench, with your hands next to your butt. Slide your butt off the edge of the bench and bend your elbows, shooting them straight back and lowering yourself until your upper arms are almost parallel to the floor. Straighten your arms and repeat.

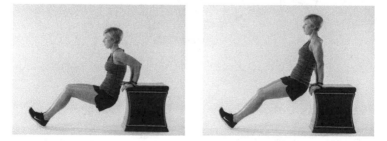

Round 3: Step Up (Right Leg)
Works your quads, hamstrings, and glutes

Stand with your right foot on the bench and your left foot on the floor behind it. Lift your left knee up, balancing on your right leg, then touch it back on the ground and immediately shoot it back up. Keep your right foot on the bench throughout.

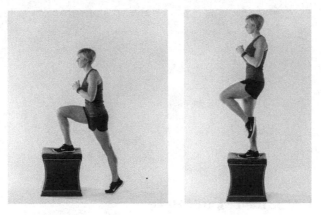

Round 4: Bench Push-ups
Works your quads, hamstrings, and glutes

Place your hands on the bench and walk your feet backward until your back is flat. Keep your core engaged and your back flat. Push up and down.

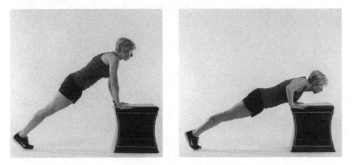

Repeat rounds 1–4.

BEGINNER TABATA #10

Round 1: Close-Stance Squat

Works your quads, hamstrings, and glutes

Stand with your feet really close together, right next to a doorjamb, pole, or railing. Hold on to the jamb and lower your body until your quads are parallel to the ground.

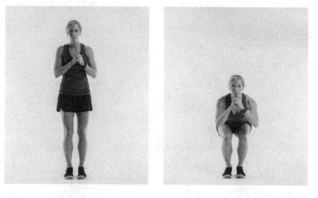

Round 2: Modified Skater Hops

Works your quads, hamstrings, hip flexors, and glutes

Squat down on your right leg, digging your left toe at an angle behind you on the ground. Hop into the same position on your other side, squatting on your left leg and digging your right toe tap at an angle behind you.

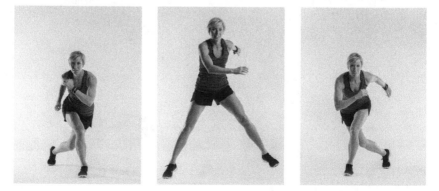

Round 3: Sumo Squat Pulses

Works your quads, hamstrings, hip flexors, and glutes

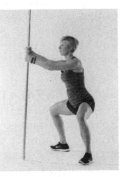

Holding on to a pole, put your feet out wide, toes turned out 45 degrees. Sink into a sumo squat and hold. Push off your heels and pulse up and down, just a few inches in each direction.

Round 4: Elevated Burpee

Cardio + works your whole body

Squat down with your hands on an ottoman, stair, or bench. Jump your feet out, keeping your back flat. Jump your feet back in, stand back up, and jump.

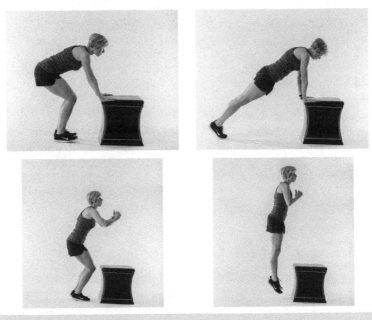

If the jumping motion is painful or impossible, try stepping out into the burpee instead of jumping. Make sure you do as much of the exercise as possible.

Repeat rounds 1–4.

BEGINNER TABATA INDEX

BEGINNER TABATA #1
Round 1: Knee Push-ups
Round 2: Floor Dips
Round 3: Right Leg Bridge Pulses
Round 4: Left Leg Bridge Pulses
Repeat rounds 1–4.

BEGINNER TABATA #2
Round 1: Jumping Jacks
Round 2: Running in Place
Round 3: Mountain Climbers
Round 4: Cross Jumping Jacks
Repeat rounds 1–4.

BEGINNER TABATA #3
Round 1: Straight Punches
Round 2: Jab Left, Cross Right
Round 3: Jab Right, Cross Left
Round 4: Hook Punches
Repeat rounds 1–4.

BEGINNER TABATA #4
Round 1: Squats
Round 2: Shoulder Presses
Round 3: Sumo Squats
Round 4: Bicep Curls
Repeat rounds 1–4.

BEGINNER TABATA #5
Round 1: Reverse Lunge Switch
Round 2: Bent-Over Rows
Round 3: High-Knee Elbow Taps
Round 4: Lateral Raises
Repeat rounds 1–4.

BEGINNER TABATA #6
Round 1: High Plank
Round 2: Knee Push-ups
Round 3: Skydivers
Round 4: Tippy-Toe Bridges
Repeat rounds 1–4.

BEGINNER TABATA #7
Round 1: Hammer Curls
Round 2: Tricep Kickbacks
Round 3: Small Arm Rotations
Round 4: V Front Raise
Repeat rounds 1–4.

BEGINNER TABATA #8
Round 1: Pretend Jump Rope
Round 2: Side Shuffle
Round 3: Windmills
Round 4: Squat Holds
Repeat rounds 1–4.

BEGINNER TABATA #9
Round 1: Step Up (Left Leg)
Round 2: Bench Dips
Round 3: Step Up (Right Leg)
Round 4: Bench Push-ups
Repeat rounds 1–4.

BEGINNER TABATA #10
Round 1: Close-Stance Squat
Round 2: Modified Skater Hops
Round 3: Sumo Squat Pulses
Round 4: Elevated Burpee
Repeat rounds 1–4.

And remember, the tabatas work like this:

Round 1:	20 seconds of exercise 10 seconds of rest	Round 5:	20 seconds of exercise 10 seconds of rest
Round 2:	20 seconds of exercise 10 seconds of rest	Round 6:	20 seconds of exercise 10 seconds of rest
Round 3:	20 seconds of exercise 10 seconds of rest	Round 7:	20 seconds of exercise 10 seconds of rest
Round 4:	20 seconds of exercise 10 seconds of rest	Round 8:	20 seconds of exercise 10 seconds of rest

INTERMEDIATE TABATAS

After doing Beginner Tabatas regularly for a while, you should reach a point where you can complete a full workout without becoming exhausted. Ideally, this will happen within two weeks. Begin incorporating Intermediate Tabatas into your routine the second you're ready for the challenge.

Like the Beginner Tabatas, many of the Intermediate Tabatas consist of four exercises that you'll perform twice. A few Intermediate Tabatas consist of two exercises that you'll perform four times each. Either way, you're still using that familiar four-minute format: eight total rounds made up of twenty seconds of intense exercise, then ten seconds of rest. These tabatas kick up the intensity—but they're still fun! (Disclaimer: my definition of "fun" may vary slightly from yours.) As a reminder, you'll know you're ready to move on to Intermediate Tabatas once you continue through the full Beginner Tabata without feeling challenged.

INTERMEDIATE TABATA #1

You'll need a jump rope for all eight rounds.

Round 1: Jump Rope
Cardio

Swing your arms forward and jump over the rope, keeping your elbows glued to your sides.

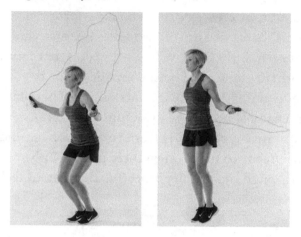

Round 2: High-Knee Jump Rope
Cardio

As you jump rope, engage your abs and pull your knees up high in front of you for the entire twenty seconds.

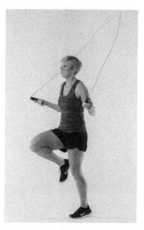

Round 3: Right Foot Jump Rope

Cardio

Hop on your right foot for the entire twenty seconds, keeping your elbows glued to your sides.

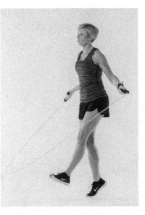

Round 4: Left Foot Jump Rope

Cardio

Hop on your left foot for the entire twenty seconds, keeping your elbows glued to your sides.

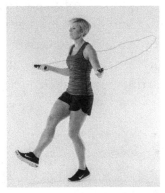

Repeat rounds 1–4.

INTERMEDIATE TABATA #2

Round 1: Reverse Lunge (Right Leg)
Works your quads, hamstrings, and glutes

Stand with your weight on your right leg. Take a large step back with your left leg and drop your left knee straight down toward the ground until your right leg is parallel to the floor, never letting your left knee hit the floor. Driving through your right heel, return to the starting position with your left knee slightly lifted.

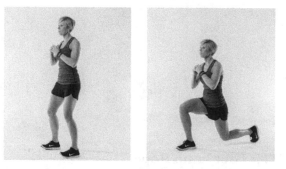

Round 2: Reverse Lunge (Left Leg)
Works your quads, hamstrings, and glutes

Stand with your weight on your left leg. Take a large step back with your right leg and drop your right knee straight down toward the ground until your left leg is parallel to the floor, never letting your right knee hit the floor. Driving through your left heel, return to the starting position with your right knee slightly lifted.

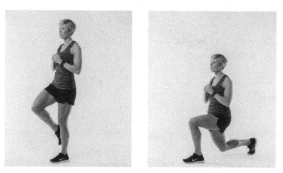

Round 3: Squats
Works your quads, hamstrings, and glutes

With your legs shoulder width apart, tilt your hips back as if you were about to sit in a chair. Lower your body until your upper legs are parallel to the floor before driving through your heels to return to the standing position.

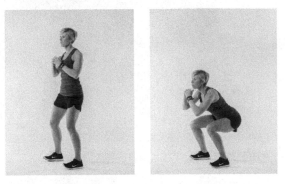

Round 4: Skater Hops
Works your quads, hamstrings, glutes, and hip flexors

Squat down on your right leg, and bend your left leg behind you at a 90-degree angle. Hop into a left leg squat and bend your left leg behind you at a 90-degree angle.

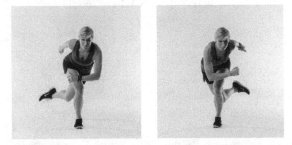

For these Skater Hops, unlike the modified version in Beginner Tabata #10, your inside foot will swing behind your squatting leg and never touch the ground before "launching" in the opposite direction.

Repeat rounds 1–4.

INTERMEDIATE TABATA #3

Round 1: Bicep Curls
Works your biceps

Hold a 5- to 10-pound weight in each hand. With your palms up and elbows glued to your sides, control the weights up and down.

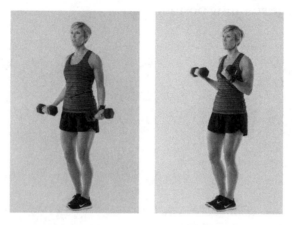

Round 2: Shoulder Presses
Works your shoulders and triceps

Stand with your arms out wide, elbows at shoulder level, and holding a 5- to 15-pound weight in each hand. Push the weights straight up and then return to shoulder level.

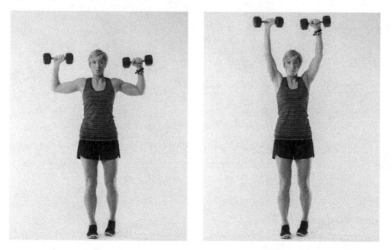

Round 3: Hammer Curls

Works your biceps

Grab a pair of 5- to 10-pound weights and grip them with your thumbs facing up. Keeping your elbows glued to your sides, curl your arms upward with your thumbs facing up.

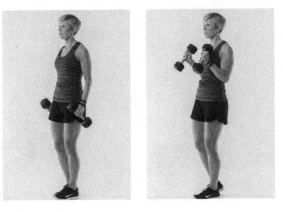

Round 4: Lateral Raises

Works your shoulders

Grab a pair of 5- to 15-pound weights, bend your elbows slightly, and keep your knees soft. Raise your arms straight out to the sides, up to shoulder level, elbows still soft. Lower to starting position.

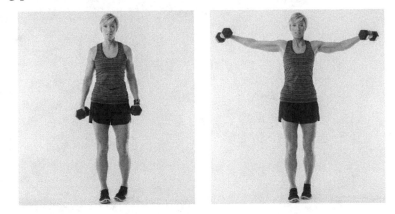

Repeat rounds 1–4.

INTERMEDIATE TABATA #4

Round 1: Bench Dips
Works your triceps

Sit on the bench, with your hands next to your butt. Slide your butt off the edge of the bench and bend your elbows, shooting them straight back and lowering yourself until your upper arms are almost parallel to the floor. Straighten your arms and repeat.

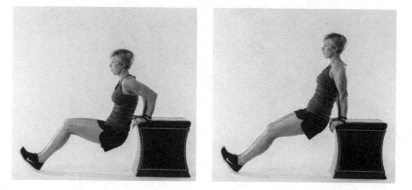

Round 2: Tricep Kickbacks
Works your triceps

Grab a pair of 5- to 10-pound weights and fall forward at your waist, with your back flat and elbows bent 90 degrees at your sides. Extend both arms straight back, squeezing your triceps. Return to starting position.

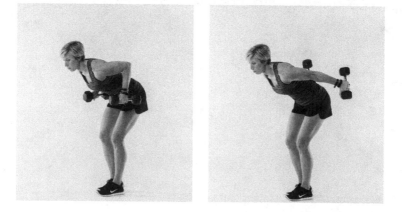

Round 3: V Front Raise
Works your shoulders

Start with your arms at your sides, holding a pair of 3- to 10-pound weights. Raise them in front of you up to shoulder level, creating a V in the air. Reverse in a controlled manner to return to starting position.

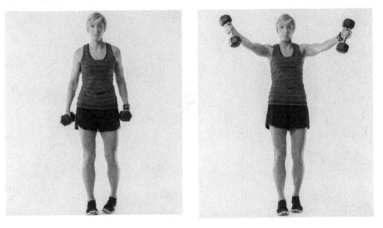

Round 4: Upright Rows
Works your shoulders and back

Stand tall and grab a pair of 5- to 10-pound weights, palms facing your thighs in front of you. Pull the weights up to your shoulders with your elbows bending out to the sides. Lower and repeat.

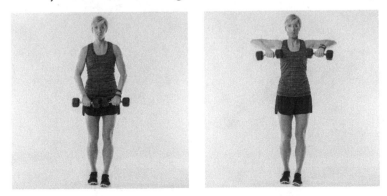

Repeat rounds 1–4.

INTERMEDIATE TABATA #5

Round 1: Jumping Lunges
Cardio + works your quads, hamstrings, and glutes

Start in a right lunge position with your right leg at a 90-degree angle and your left knee straight down and hovering just above the floor. Now drive through your right heel and jump up, switching foot placement in the air. Land softly and repeat.

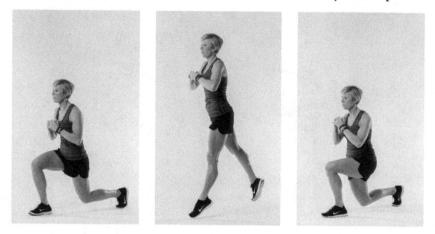

Round 2: Plank with Glute Squeeze
Works your core and glutes

Get into plank position on your hands. Hold, keeping your legs, butt, and core engaged (that's the glute squeeze).

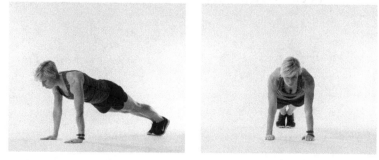

Round 3: Mountain Climbers

Cardio + works your core

Get into plank position with your back flat and hands straight below your shoulders. Keeping your core tight, bring one knee toward your chest, then take it back; switch legs. You should feel like you're running in place in prone position.

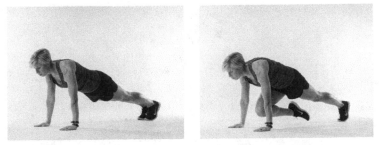

Round 4: Sumo Squat Jump and Tap

Works your inner thighs, quads, hamstrings, and glutes

Turn out your toes 45 degrees and lower your body into a sumo squat. Jump up and bring your feet together as you land, just barely tapping the ground, then jump back out into the sumo squat position.

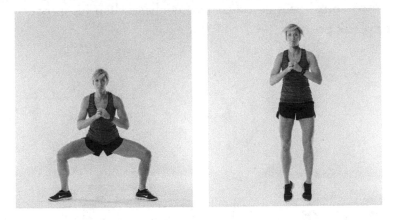

Repeat rounds 1–4.

INTERMEDIATE TABATA #6

Round 1: Push-ups
Works your chest and core
Get into plank position, with your hands slightly wider than your shoulders. Lower your body toward the floor until your elbows are at 90 degrees. Push back to starting position. Keep your core engaged the entire time.

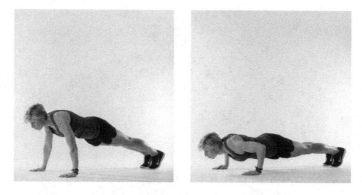

Round 2: Plank In-and-Outs
Cardio + works your core and shoulders
Start in a plank position on your hands and toes, with your back flat, core engaged, and feet together. Jump both feet forward so your knees go toward your chest, then jump back out into plank position.

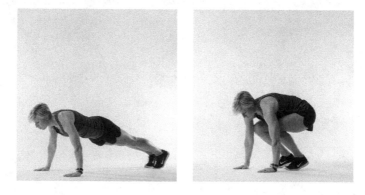

Repeat rounds 1 and 2 four times.

INTERMEDIATE TABATA #7

Round 1: Squats
Works your quads, hamstrings, and glutes

Place your feet shoulder width apart and squat low until your legs are parallel to the ground. Keep your weight on your heels and your chest up.

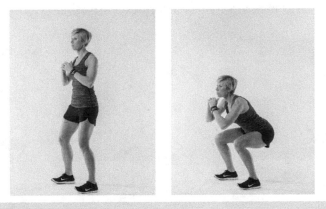

Proper form is everything here—maintain it!

Round 2: Sumo Squats
Works your quads, inner thighs, and glutes

Place your feet wider than shoulder width apart and turn out your toes 45 degrees. Push your butt out as if you were sitting on a chair and lower your body until your legs are parallel to the ground. Dig through your heels and stand back up.

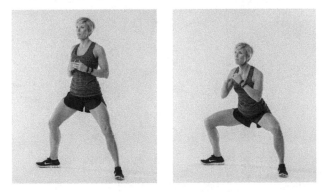

Repeat rounds 1 and 2 four times.

INTERMEDIATE TABATA #8

Round 1: Burpees
Cardio + works your whole body

Perform a push-up, then hop your feet in toward your arms, drive up through a squat, and jump into the air. As you return to the ground, immediately lower into a squat, place your hands on the floor, and kick your legs back out for another push-up.

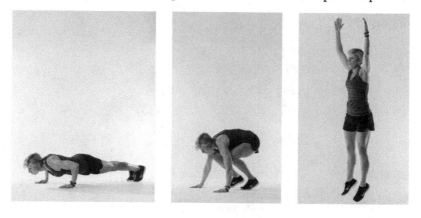

Round 2: Jumping Jacks
Cardio

Stand upright with your feet together and your arms by your sides. Jump and land with your feet shoulder width apart, simultaneously raising your arms overhead. Jump back to starting position.

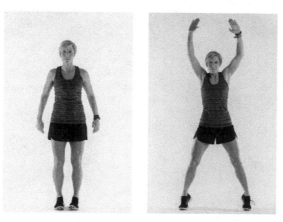

Round 3: Squat Jumps
Works your quads, hams, and glutes

Stand with your feet shoulder width apart, chest up, and weight on your heels. Squat until your legs are parallel to the ground. Now jump into the air, land softly, and repeat immediately.

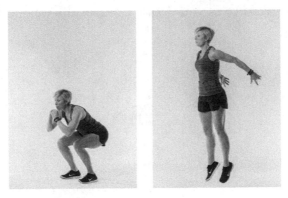

Round 4: High Knees
Cardio

Run in place, bringing each knee up in front of your body and keeping your core tight.

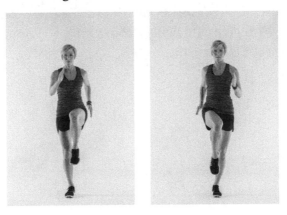

Repeat rounds 1–4.

INTERMEDIATE TABATA #9

Round 1: Reverse Fly
Works your back and shoulders

Stand with a 5- to 15-pound weight in each hand and a slight bend in your knees. Fall forward at the waist, keeping your back flat. Now, with a slight bend in your elbows, bring your arms out wide until they are parallel to the ground, squeezing your shoulder blades together as you do so. Control the weight down and repeat.

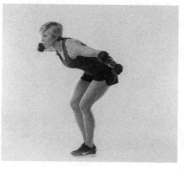

Round 2: Push-ups
Works your chest, triceps, and core

Get into plank position, with your hands slightly wider than your shoulders. Lower your body toward the floor until your elbows are at 90 degrees. Push back to starting position. Keep your core engaged the entire time.

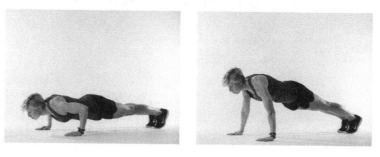

Round 3: V Front Raise
Works your shoulders

Start with your arms at your sides, holding a pair of 3- to 10-pound weights. Raise them in front of you up to shoulder level, creating a V in the air. Reverse in a controlled manner to return to starting position.

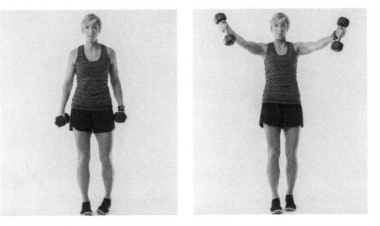

Round 4: Military Push-ups
Works your triceps, core, chest, and shoulders

Place your hands below your shoulders with your back and abs engaged. Bend your arms, elbows going straight back against your ribs, and lower your body until your elbows form 90 degrees and then push up from this position. Don't let your back sag!

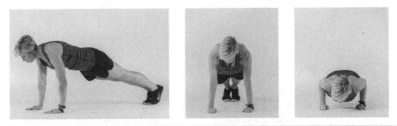

During push-ups, you can drop to your knees if you need to—the key is to keep going.

Repeat rounds 1–4.

INTERMEDIATE TABATA #10

Round 1: Side Lunge Right

Works your quads, hamstrings, glutes, and inner thighs

Take a big step to the right, putting the majority of your weight on your right heel, and lower your body until your right leg is parallel to the ground. Keep your left leg straight. Push through your right heel, driving your right knee up in front of you. Repeat on same leg.

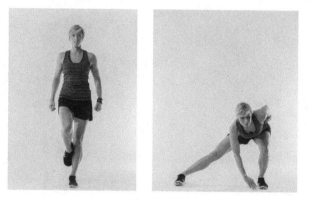

Round 2: Side Lunge Left

Works your quads, hamstrings, glutes, and inner thighs

Take a big step to the left, putting the majority of your weight on your left heel, and lower your body until your left leg is parallel to the ground. Keep your right leg straight. Push through your left heel, driving your left knee up in front of you. Repeat on same leg.

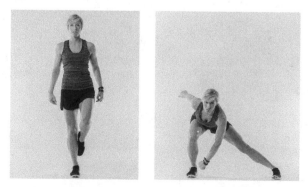

Round 3: Elbow Plank with Hip Dip
Works your core and obliques

Get into plank position, resting on your elbows. Rotate your hips downward and dip them to the left side, then back up to center. Then rotate your hips downward to the right, then back up to center. Keep the rest of your body still the entire time.

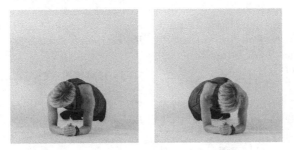

Round 4: V-Up Hold
Works your core

Lie on your back, with your arms straight out and legs straight and together. Bring your shoulders off ground with your arms extended up, to meet legs off the ground. Create a V with your body and hold as long as you can.

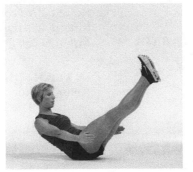

Repeat rounds 1–4.

BONUS INTERMEDIATE TABATAS

Rounds 1–8: Push-ups
Rounds 1–8: Floor Dips

INTERMEDIATE TABATA INDEX

INTERMEDIATE TABATA #1
Round 1: Jump Rope
Round 2: High-Knee Jump Rope
Round 3: Right Foot Jump Rope
Round 4: Left Foot Jump Rope
Repeat rounds 1–4.

INTERMEDIATE TABATA #2
Round 1: Reverse Lunge (Right
     Leg)
Round 2: Reverse Lunge (Left Leg)
Round 3: Squats
Round 4: Skater Hops
Repeat rounds 1–4.

INTERMEDIATE TABATA #3
Round 1: Bicep Curls
Round 2: Shoulder Presses
Round 3: Hammer Curls
Round 4: Lateral Raises
Repeat rounds 1–4.

INTERMEDIATE TABATA #4
Round 1: Bench Dips
Round 2: Tricep Kickbacks
Round 3: V Front Raise
Round 4: Upright Rows
Repeat rounds 1–4.

INTERMEDIATE TABATA #5
Round 1: Jumping Lunges
Round 2: Plank with Glute Squeeze
Round 3: Mountain Climbers
Round 4: Sumo Squat Jump and
     Tap
Repeat rounds 1–4.

INTERMEDIATE TABATA #6
Round 1: Push-ups
Round 2: Plank In-and-Outs
Repeat rounds 1 and 2 four times.

INTERMEDIATE TABATA #7
Round 1: Squats
Round 2: Sumo Squats
Repeat rounds 1 and 2 four times.

INTERMEDIATE TABATA #8
Round 1: Burpees
Round 2: Jumping Jacks
Round 3: Squat Jumps
Round 4: High Knees
Repeat rounds 1–4.

INTERMEDIATE TABATA #9
Round 1: Reverse Fly
Round 2: Push-ups
Round 3: V Front Raise
Round 4: Military Push-ups
Repeat rounds 1–4.

INTERMEDIATE TABATA #10
Round 1: Side Lunge Right
Round 2: Side Lunge Left
Round 3: Elbow Plank with Hip
     Dip
Round 4: V-Up Hold
Repeat rounds 1–4.

**BONUS INTERMEDIATE
     TABATAS**
Rounds 1–8: Push-ups
Rounds 1–8: Floor Dips

ADVANCED TABATAS

You'll notice that a couple of these Advanced Tabatas consist of only one move, which you'll repeat for all eight rounds. That is the hardest tabata variation, since you're working the exact same muscles for nearly four minutes straight. The other moves in this group are also harder compared to the Beginner and Intermediate Tabatas; all ten of these will test your strength, balance, and endurance. But you've worked so hard to get up to this point—and I know you'll be able to master all of them when you're ready. You'll know you're ready to move on to the Advanced Tabatas once you continue through the full Intermediate Tabatas without feeling challenged.

ADVANCED TABATA #1

Rounds 1–4: Squat into Left Lunge
Works your quads, hamstrings, and glutes

Squat down on your left leg, right toes lightly touching the floor for balance. Without standing up, take your right leg back into a lunge. Keep your left leg bent and return your right leg to starting position.

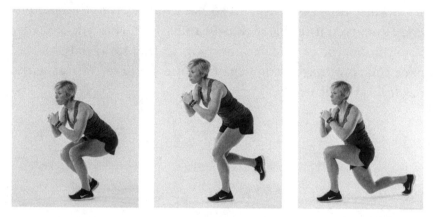

Rounds 5–8: Squat into Right Lunge
Works your quads, hamstrings, and glutes

Squat down on your right leg, left toes lightly touching the floor for balance. Without standing up, take your left leg back into a lunge. Keep your right leg bent and return your left leg to starting position.

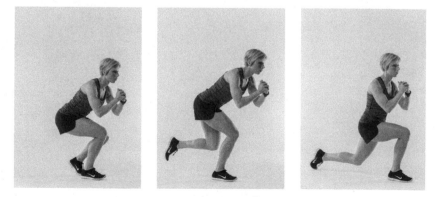

ADVANCED TABATA #2

Round 1: Left Leg V-Up Claps
Works your core

Lie on your back with your legs extended straight on the floor. Raise your left leg and upper body to form a V. Clap under your left leg before returning to starting position.

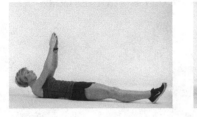 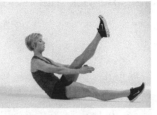

Round 2: Right Leg V-Up Claps
Works your core

Lie on your back with your legs extended straight on the floor. Raise your right leg and upper body to form a V. Clap under your right leg before returning to starting position.

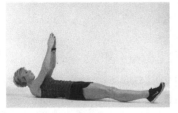 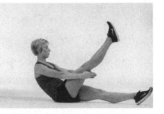

Alternate these two moves for eight rounds.

ADVANCED TABATA #3

Round 1: Burpees
Cardio + works your whole body

Perform a push-up, then hop your feet in toward your arms, drive up through a squat, and jump into the air. As you return to the ground, immediately lower into a squat, place your hands on the floor, and kick your legs back out for another push-up.

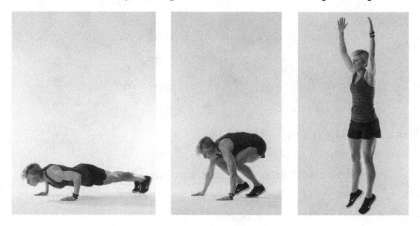

Round 2: Squat into Shoulder Press
Works your quads, hamstrings, glutes, and shoulders

Hold a pair of 5- to 15-pound dumbbells at your shoulders and perform a squat. Once you stand back up, press the weights above your head. Lower and return to starting position.

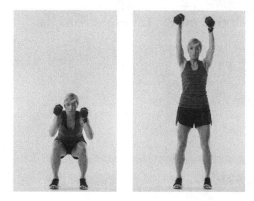

Alternate these two moves for eight rounds.

ADVANCED TABATA #4

Rounds 1–8: Mountain Climbers with Plank
Cardio + works your core

Get into plank position with your back flat and hands straight below your shoulders. Keeping your core tight, bring one knee toward your chest, then take it back; switch legs. Here's the twist: After each set of mountain climbers, stay in plank position instead of resting.

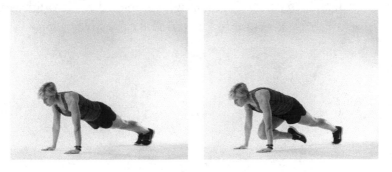

ADVANCED TABATA #5

For curtsy lunges, keep your hips facing forward at all times.
For added difficulty, place your stationary foot on a step.

Rounds 1–4: Curtsy Lunges (Right Leg)
Works your hips, quads, and "saddlebags"

Lunge back with your right leg, crossing it behind your left leg (as if you were doing a dramatic curtsy). Bend both knees until your left leg forms a 90-degree angle. Then drive through your left heel and lift your right leg, balancing on your left leg.

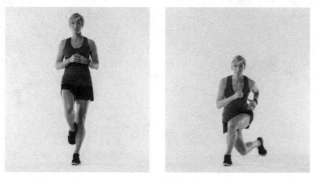

Rounds 5–8: Curtsy Lunges (Left Leg)
Works your hips, quads, and "saddlebags"

Lunge back with your left leg, crossing it behind your right leg (as if you were doing a dramatic curtsy). Bend both knees until your right leg forms a 90-degree angle. Then drive through your right heel and lift your left leg, balancing on your right leg.

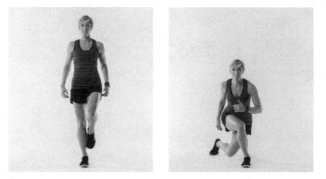

ADVANCED TABATA #6

Round 1: 180-Degree Jump Squats
Cardio + works your quads and glutes

Perform a jumping squat, rotating your entire body 180 degrees while in the air. Keep rotating in the same direction so you jump left, then right.

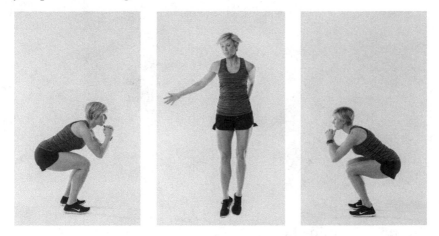

Round 2: Sumo Squat Jumps with Air Tap
Works your inner thighs, quads, and glutes

Lower into a sumo squat, then jump up and quickly tap your feet together in the air before going wide again with your feet. Land in a sumo squat.

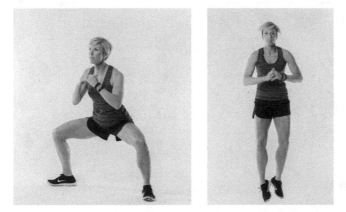

Round 3: Downhill Ski Hops

Cardio + works your quads and glutes

Stand with your feet close together, and squat as if you were on skis. Jump side to side, keeping your feet close together.

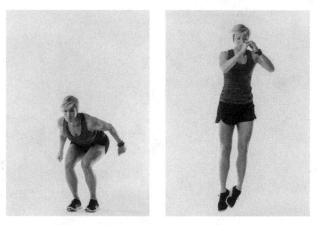

Round 4: Jumping Lunges

Works your glutes, quads, and hamstrings

Start in a right lunge position, with your right leg at a 90-degree angle and your left knee straight down and hovering just above the floor. Now drive through your right heel and jump up, switching foot placement in the air. Land softly and repeat.

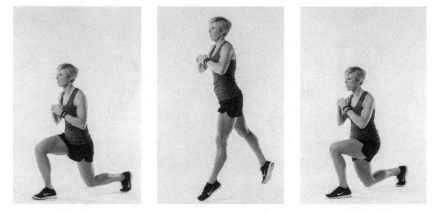

Repeat rounds 1–4.

ADVANCED TABATA #7

Rounds 1–4: One-Legged Squat Jumps (Right Leg)
Works your quads, hamstrings, and glutes

Stand on your right leg, floating your left leg behind you, and squat with your right leg. As you stand up, drive your left knee forward and up and hop on your right leg. Land and return to starting position.

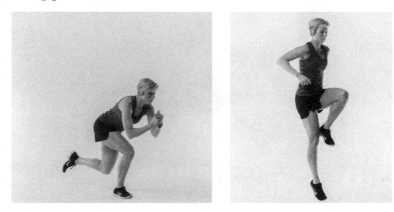

Rounds 5–8: One-Legged Squat Jumps (Left Leg)
Works your quads, hamstrings, and glutes

Stand on your left leg, floating your right leg behind you, and squat with your left leg. As you stand up, drive your right knee forward and up and hop on your left leg. Land and return to starting position.

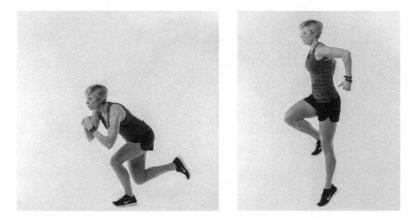

ADVANCED TABATA #8

Round 1: Right Side Elbow Plank
Works your obliques and core

Get into a plank on your right side, elbow on the floor and lined up with your right shoulder. Stack your feet, push your hips up, and engage your core. Hold.

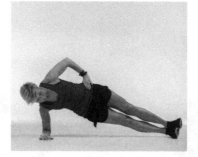

Round 2: Left Side Elbow Plank
Works your obliques and core

Get into a plank on your left side, elbow on the floor and lined up with your left shoulder. Stack your feet, push your hips up, and engage your core. Hold.

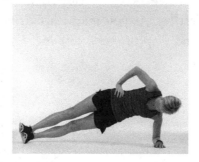

Round 3: Plank Up-Downs, Starting on Left
Works your shoulders, chest, and core

Start in a plank on your hands. Lower your left elbow down onto the mat, then lower your right elbow down onto the mat. Lift yourself back up to starting plank position.

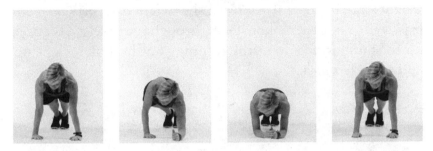

Round 4: Plank Up-Downs, Starting on Right
Works your shoulders, chest, and core

Start in a plank on your hands. Lower your right elbow down onto the mat, then lower your left elbow down onto the mat. Lift yourself back up to starting plank position.

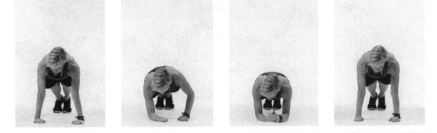

For Plank Up-Downs, don't let your body sway from side to side as you maneuver up and down.

Repeat rounds 1–4.

ADVANCED TABATA #9

Round 1: Cherry Pickers
Works your hamstrings

Hold a 20- to 40-pound dumbbell with both hands. Stand with your legs wide and knees softened. Bend at the hips—keeping your back flat, chest up, and shoulders back—as you lower the weight straight down. Then reach the weight back between your legs, controlling the motion. Push through your heels to lift back up to standing position, still keeping your back flat, chest up, and shoulders back.

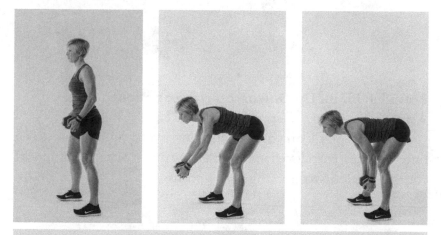

Cherry Pickers call for a single heavy dumbbell, but you can swap it out for a similarly weighted kettlebell—it may be easier to grip for this move and any others that involve slow, controlled movements. I prefer dumbbells because they can do everything a kettlebell can do, and then some.

Round 2: Frog Jumps

Cardio + works your quads, glutes, and hamstrings

Squat down, touch the ground, and jump forward.

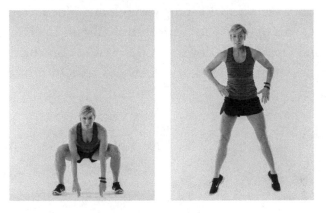

Repeat four times.

ADVANCED TABATA #10

Rounds 1–8: Hammer Curls with Military Push-ups
Works your whole body

Grab a pair of 10- to 15-pound weights and grip them with your thumbs facing up. Keeping your elbows glued to your sides, curl your arms upward with your thumbs facing up. During each ten-second "rest," drop down, set the weights on the floor, and grip them as you do Military Push-ups (see Intermediate Tabata #9 on page 172).

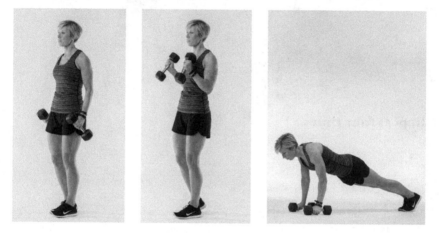

ADVANCED TABATA INDEX

ADVANCED TABATA #1
Rounds 1–4: Squat into Left Lunge
Rounds 5–8: Squat into Right
      Lunge

ADVANCED TABATA #2
Round 1: Left Leg V-Up Claps
Round 2: Right Leg V-Up Claps
*Alternate these two moves for eight
      rounds.*

ADVANCED TABATA #3
Round 1: Burpees
Round 2: Squat into Shoulder Press
*Alternate these two moves for eight
      rounds.*

ADVANCED TABATA #4
Rounds 1–8: Mountain Climbers
      with Plank

ADVANCED TABATA #5
Rounds 1–4: Curtsy Lunges, Right
      Leg
Rounds 5–8: Curtsy Lunges, Left
      Leg

ADVANCED TABATA #6
Round 1: 180-Degree Jump Squats
Round 2: Sumo Squat Jumps with
      Air Tap
Round 3: Downhill Ski Hops
Round 4: Jumping Lunges
Repeat rounds 1–4.

ADVANCED TABATA #7
Rounds 1–4: One-Legged Squat
      Jumps, Right Leg
Rounds 5–8: One-Legged Squat
      Jumps, Left Leg

ADVANCED TABATA #8
Round 1: Right Side Elbow Plank
Round 2: Left Side Elbow Plank
Round 3: Plank Up-Downs,
      Starting on Left
Round 4: Plank Up-Downs,
      Starting on Right
Repeat rounds 1–4.

ADVANCED TABATA #9
Round 1: Cherry Pickers
Round 2: Frog Jumps
Repeat four times.

ADVANCED TABATA #10
Rounds 1–8: Hammer Curls with
      Military Push-ups

CHAPTER 13

Tabata Variations and Modifications

CARDIO TABATAS

Let's not forget that the original tabata workouts done by the Japanese speed skaters consisted of eight consecutive rounds of high-intensity cardio. With that in mind, try these treadmill- and stationary bike–based tabatas and push yourself to the max in every round. If you're not fully exhausted by the time the four minutes is up, then you need to crank up the intensity.

CARDIO TABATA #1

Rounds 1–8: Set the treadmill to between 6 and 12 mph and keep it at that speed for the entire exercise. Sprint for twenty seconds, then jump to the side of the treadmill and rest for ten seconds while the treadmill continues to run. Jump back on and repeat.

CARDIO TABATA #2

Round 1: Set the treadmill speed between 6 and 12 mph. Sprint for twenty seconds, then rest for ten seconds.
Round 2: Slow down the treadmill speed to between 3 and 5.5

mph. Run backward for twenty seconds, then rest for ten seconds.

Repeat rounds 1 and 2 four times.

CARDIO TABATA #3

Rounds 1–8: Set the treadmill to an incline of 7 and set the speed anywhere from 5 to 8 mph. Hold on and jump off carefully during rest time.

CARDIO TABATA #4

Rounds 1–8: Set the treadmill to an incline between 6 and 10 and walk at 3.3 to 4.2 mph, depending on your level. Hold on and jump off carefully during rest time.

CARDIO TABATA #5

Rounds 1–8: Crank up the resistance on a spin bike and pedal as fast as you can for twenty seconds. Turn down the resistance and rest for ten seconds.

OTHER WAYS TO MODIFY TABATAS

I've already mentioned that tabata has great flexibility—you can apply all kinds of moves to the tabata format. In fact, of the thirty tabatas I've just shown you, only a few of the moves, like push-ups and dips, are repeated in multiple tabatas. It's important to vary the moves you perform throughout the days and weeks so that you don't hit a plateau physically as well as mentally. To avoid that rut, you should be constantly challenging your body and your mind.

Thanks to the following modifications, tabatas become even more flexible, meaning it's even easier to come up with ways to challenge yourself. When you apply the following tweaks to your favorite exercises (or even your not-so-favorite exercises), you'll see why you never have to do the exact same workout twice. With tabatas, the possibilities are truly endless.

Modification #1: You can change up the number of exercises.

All tabatas consist of eight rounds. Many of the tabatas I've shown you consist of four different exercises, each of which you perform twice. Others, like Intermediate Tabata #7, consist of two moves, which you perform four times each. This modification makes the tabata harder since you're working the same muscle groups twice as much. And in Advanced Tabata #4, you perform just one move—in this case, mountain climbers with a plank—eight times in a row. This modification makes the tabata harder still, since you're using the same muscle groups even *more*, with minimal breaks. In both of these modifications, you still end up with eight rounds.

Because there are eight rounds, you can do:
- 1 move 8 times
- 2 moves 4 times
- 4 moves 2 times

Modification #2: You can add weights to nonweighted exercises—or more weight to weighted exercises.

Any move that requires dumbbells or kettlebells can be made more challenging by upping the amount of weight. For example, Intermediate Tabata #9 calls for two rounds of reverse flies, where you shoot your arms out to the sides while holding a pair of dumbbells. Start with 5 pounds the first few times you do this move. After a few workouts where you incorporate reverse flies, which may take several weeks if you're really mixing up your tabatas, you should find 5 pounds to be easy. When that happens, bump up the weight to 8 pounds. When that weight becomes comfortable, bump it up again to 10 pounds, and so on. The same rule applies to curls, shoulder presses, punches, squats, and more.

It's important to note that just because you are able to lift heavier weights, that doesn't mean that you aren't allowed to go back down to a lower weight. Starting out heavier to challenge yourself may very well lead to ending the tabata at a lighter weight. When your form starts to falter, lower the weights so that you still get the most out of the exercise. Just don't stop moving—or maintaining correct form.

Modification #3: You can keep moving during the rest period.

To make any move harder, turn the ten seconds of rest into active rest. You can:

- Run in place
- Do jumping jacks
- Do high knees
- Do butt kicks
- Drop and hold a plank, engaging your core

Modification #4: You can change the timing of the tabata itself.

The tabata format is twenty seconds of intense exercise, then ten seconds of rest—this follows the original tabata study of male college students on stationary bikes, and it's the ratio I use most frequently myself and with clients. But if you're looking for a challenge, you can adjust the tabata timer to make the periods of exercise and rest even longer. Example: when you're doing planks, make the "work" timer last for one minute and the "rest" period last thirty seconds. You can do eight rounds or even push it to ten rounds. On the flip side, if you're just starting out or nursing an injury, you can knock it down to four or even two rounds if necessary.

Modification #5: You can break up your tabata workout.

Finally, there's one aspect of tabatas that not all other workouts can claim: if you don't have a solid thirty- or forty-five-minute block to devote to a complete workout, you can break it up into four-minute workouts throughout your day. While it's ideal to do all four to six tabatas in a row, in one session, you don't necessarily have to. On days when you're on the go nonstop, fit these four-minute exercises into any ten-minute pockets of downtime: knock out two tabatas as you're brewing coffee in the morning, two more before lunch, and two more while you watch the evening news. *That's* how you squeeze a good workout into your busy day.

CHAPTER 14

Exercises for Injuries and Ailments

The following exercises are suggestions for minor ailments only. For example, follow the sore shoulder guidelines if you slept on it wrong—rather than if you're recovering from shoulder surgery. As always, check with your physician before performing any of these exercises. You don't want to risk making an existing condition worse.

A sore knee or ankle

Sore knees could be caused by a sudden, sharp increase in normal activities, such as extra pickup basketball games or going up and down stairs more than usual (say you're moving out of your house). They may also be caused by carrying excess weight—an unfortunate catch-22 when you're trying to get lean, but some discomfort is to be expected when working out. If you put a hyperfocus on correct form while working out your legs, it can alleviate the pain.

- **Seated boxing.** Boxing is a great exercise whether you're standing up or sitting down. Pull up a chair to a boxing bag and go at it—engaging your core for extra stability and added difficulty—and you'll get your heart rate up in no time.

- **Rope pull-down machine.** Many gyms have Nautilus machines that help you sculpt your upper body and scorch calories. This was my go-to machine after my MCL and ACL surgeries.
- **Arm exercises with dumbbells.** Don't forget about all the weighted upper-body moves you can do while seated: shoulder presses, arm curls, overhead tricep extensions, lateral raises—basically, any moves you normally do standing.

A sore back

- **Stretching.** An achy back may be the result of tight hamstrings, and stretching can do wonders. Also try grabbing a foam roller and rolling out your lower back as well as your hips and hamstrings.
- **Bird dogs and skydivers.** These are my favorite moves for strengthening your back and core.

Bird dogs: Get on your hands and knees, and with your butt squeezed, stretch out your right arm and left leg so both are parallel to the ground. Then pull them back in toward your body, bringing your right elbow to your left knee and tucking your belly button into your spine. Perform ten to fifteen reps before switching to the opposite arm and leg: That's one set; repeat that two or three times.

Skydivers: Lie on your stomach and rotate your arms to your side with your palms up. Pull your chest and quads up off the ground simultaneously. Now drop your head down to keep the pressure off your neck (see page 147 for a visual). As the name implies, it should look like you're skydiving. Try to hold for fifteen to twenty seconds. Aim for two or three rounds to strengthen your back.

- **Stabilizer ball wall squats.** Place a big stabilizer ball against a wall and lean back against the ball. With the ball supporting your back, you can perform lots of basic moves with light weights: curls, shoulder presses, lateral raises.

One of my clients who has a long history of back pain loves this move so much that I can see his delight every time I pull out the stability ball. It feels *that* good on his back.

- **Recumbent biking.** On this machine, your back is supported and the cardio will keep your heart strong.

A sore shoulder

- **Leg and core exercises.** Now's a great opportunity to mix in some hamstring exercises. Get your heart pumping with lunge and squat variations, bicycle crunches, or hamstring curls on a stability ball.
- **Lightweight upper-body exercises.** Grab a lighter pair of dumbbells than you usually use and knock out a few sets of bicep curls and hammer curls.

A sore wrist or elbow

- **Leg and core exercises.** Again, use this as an opportunity to play up lunges and squat variations.
- **Your favorite form of cardio.** Running, stair-climbing, hip-hop dancing . . .
- **Assisted push-ups.** If you have minor soreness in your wrist and/or have difficulty bending it, minimize the pressure you put on it with a set of Perfect Pushup handles. One of my clients can't do regular push-ups on the ground due to a fall in the past, but he does great with these rubberized grips. A set should cost about $30.

A cold or allergies

If you're not running a fever and don't have chest congestion, try doing a lighter, less intense version of your regular workout:

jogging instead of running, fewer reps, or fewer sets. This will almost always make you feel much better than just lying around. Once you motivate yourself to take that first step out the door into the fresh air, the hardest part is over. Keep in mind: you don't have to put in 100 percent when you're not feeling 100 percent. Expending energy will still magically make you feel like you have more energy.

Bunions

These bulging, burning-sensation bumps at the base of the big toe can be caused by wearing narrow shoes or having prior foot injuries; they're also thought to be inherited. Unfortunately, the only way to get rid of them is through surgery. If you're dealing with an inflamed bunion, you'll want to avoid moves that involve pushing off or jumping off the affected foot. When it comes to leg exercises, your best bet is to stick with moves where both of your feet remain on the ground, like squats.

Stomachache or menstrual cramps

Stomachaches are tricky. Personally, I rarely work out when I have a stomachache that includes nausea—especially if I have a bug and know I may be throwing up in the near future. A lot of times this is also accompanied by a fever, which is another reason I give myself and my clients a pass.

However, ladies, if the stomach pain is stemming from your period, force yourself to get moving—even if it's just a quick walk. Moving around can relieve cramps (some experts say this is because aerobic activity releases endorphins, aka your brain's feel-good chemicals) and at the very least will take your mind off the pain.

Constipation

Movement of any kind is one of the best things to do when you're backed up—even though all you want to do is curl up in a ball. Ready for a gross-but-true motto? "Body movement will lead to bowel movement." Shoot for a ten- to fifteen-minute walk.

Exhaustion

I can't count how many times I have heard the words "I'm too tired to work out." But what exactly does that mean? You need to ask yourself if you are *sleepy* or if you are *sleep deprived*, the latter of which can lead to exhaustion.

You may be sleep deprived if you aren't getting six to eight hours of sleep each night. This is when your body recovers from everything you've put it through during the day and when it rests up so it can function properly the next day. If you are running on fewer than six hours of sleep, you need to prioritize your sleep schedule. Get back on track and pick up your workout routine as soon as possible.

On the other hand, if you're getting enough sleep and are just having an off day where you're feeling tired or sluggish, I have three words for you: *Get over it.* You've got to push through it and get yourself moving. Start by walking, doing jumping jacks, or jumping rope. Once your heart rate is up, the tiredness will fade. Need proof? I've never had a client fall asleep while we were working out. Ever.

Lightheadedness

Dizzy spells, messed-up balance, nausea—I see this a lot when I'm training clients, and it's usually because they haven't eaten (or haven't eaten the right food) before their workout. If your lightheadedness overpowers your body, sit down immediately and wait for it to pass. Don't attempt to work out again until the feeling has completely subsided.

And next time, be prepared. Every body is different, but you'll want to have a small snack anywhere from a half hour to an hour and a half before exercising. My go-to is one serving of oatmeal (that's a half cup), which gives me about 150 calories, more than 5 grams of protein, and less than 1 gram of sugar. Being dehydrated is also a common culprit, so make sure you drink water before, during, and after your workout.

PART 4

THE 4 × 4 DIET

Now it's time to take everything you've learned about the clean and lean lifestyle and put it into action. But I would never just send you off without a plan. For starters, you'll likely be making huge changes to the only diet you've ever known, so I'll show you how to roll them out gradually. And if the tabata style is completely new to you, the first step is mastering the Beginner Tabatas; once you do that, you can move on to the Intermediate and Advanced Tabatas.

All of this can be done in just four weeks. Each week, you'll incorporate a new clean eating habit and slightly more challenging tabatas. And each week, you'll feel cleaner, leaner, healthier, and stronger. That momentum will keep you going not just for four weeks straight but for the rest of your life.

Before you jump in, let's go over a few ground rules for getting clean and lean:

Clean

- *Five meals a day:* Every day, you should be eating five times: breakfast, midmorning snack, lunch, afternoon snack, and dinner. Use the 4 × 4 Recipes as you're starting out, since they were designed to ease you into the four clean eating habits, and don't forget about all the modifications and substitutions available. (The 4 × 4 Recipes begin on page 75; modifications are on page 107.) For those of you who like to see what the plan will look like in action, I've put together a twenty-eight-day sample eating plan to help you get started. If you are someone who'd rather not follow a specific plan, feel free to use all the general guidelines I've shared throughout the book to incorporate the necessary 4 × 4 changes into your current lifestyle.

·   *Combine protein and carbs:* At every meal, you should be eating a complex carbohydrate and a protein; this is your friendly reminder that complex carbs in the evening should be veggies, not grains. For example:

Breakfast: eggs + oatmeal or avocado on whole-wheat/ Ezekiel bread

Lunch: chicken + whole-wheat wrap

Dinner: zucchini noodles + tilapia

Snack: apple + peanut butter or veggies + hummus

This will keep your blood sugar from spiking and then crashing. At dinner, your complex carb should be non-starchy because you're less likely to be active after dinner. Your body won't use that starchy energy and instead might store it as the very fat you're trying to shed.

·   *Water, water, water:* You should also be taking in lots of water—remember that the goal is to drink half your body weight in ounces each day.

·   *Cheating is allowed:* And don't forget that you're allowed to indulge yourself at one meal or two per week. These "off-duty" experiences should be planned ahead of time and savored in the moment—don't blow it on an impulse food or drink you don't even enjoy.

Lean

- *Tabata workouts:* Do a tabata workout three or four times every week, with each consisting of four to six tabatas. (Beginner Tabatas start on page 134.) Ideally, you'll knock them out at once. But because these workouts last only four minutes, you can squeeze them in at different spots throughout the day (e.g., two in the morning, one right before lunch, two after work) when you're busier than usual.
- *Walk it off:* Every day, you should also be walking as much as you can, with the goal of 10,000 steps, or about five miles. Use a fitness tracker to keep track of your progress and to motivate yourself to increase that number daily.
- *Cardio can help:* Try to do thirty minutes of cardio on the days you are not doing tabatas—this is a great way to achieve those 10,000 daily steps.

You don't have to start the 4 × 4 Diet on the first day of the month or a certain day of the week. Here's my recommendation: start tomorrow.

WEEK 1:
Beginner Tabatas + Cutting Out Starches at Night

Start out strong and confident, and not just because this is the easiest week. You're now taking control of everything you put into your body, and you're testing its physical capabilities in new ways.

CLEAN

Week 1 objective: *Cut out starches at night*

- Eat all of your starches before 4 p.m.
- Make sure they're the *right* starches: whole grains and starchy veggies like sweet potatoes.
- Find nonstarchy alternatives for after lunch and dinner, like Zucchini Noodles (see page 93) and Mashed Cauliflower (see page 96).
- Keep it simple in the beginning! Grilled chicken, salmon, and tilapia are all easy, filling dinners to ease you into the clean lifestyle.

Add These to Your Grocery List:

For Breakfast and Lunch:

Brown rice	Quinoa
Hummus	Sweet potatoes
Low-sugar cereal, like Cheerios	Whole-wheat bread
	Whole-wheat pasta
Oatmeal (old-fashioned or steel-cut oats)	Whole-wheat wraps

For Dinner:

Almonds	Cauliflower
Broccoli	Chicken breasts and tenders
Brussels sprouts	Cod

Kale and/or romaine lettuce   Squash
Lean steak/red meats   Tilapia
Salmon fillets   Zucchini

Remove These from Your Grocery List:
Frozen meals
Iceberg lettuce
White bread products
White rice

Try These Dinners:
Grilled chicken with Mashed Cauliflower (see page 96)
Grilled salmon with Roasted Asparagus (see page 97)
Lettuce Wrap Tacos (see page 95)
Zucchini Noodles with Pesto and Tilapia (see page 93)
Lemon Pepper Cod (see page 93)
Lasagna Spaghetti Squash Casserole (see page 88)
Chicken Caprese (see page 94)

LEAN

Week 1 objective: *Do at least three tabata workouts, each consisting of four to six Beginner Tabatas*

· It's okay to repeat tabatas as you get the hang of the style.

BEGINNER WORKOUT PLAN

Start here, no matter your fitness level. These days are inter-changeable—if you need to knock out two workout days in a row, then do it! If you have time for only two tabatas in the morning, get the other two done in the evening. The key is to get going and keep going. You got this.

Monday

Get your steps! Today, find out what your average step count is with your tracker. Your eventual daily goal: 10,000 steps.

4 TABATAS
Warm-up
Beginner Tabata #2
Beginner Tabata #1
Beginner Tabata #4
Beginner Tabata #8
Cooldown with walking, stretching, and rolling

Tuesday

Take at least 1,000 more steps than you did yesterday.

You very well may be sore today, so take this easier cardio workout. Keep in mind that action spurs action and laziness breeds laziness!

5 minutes of casual walking warm-up
2 minutes of speed walking
2 minutes of casual walking
Repeat this for 5 rounds
5-minute cooldown session (includes stretching and foam rolling)

Friday

Match the steps that you took yesterday!

4 TABATAS
Warm-up
Beginner Tabata #9
Beginner Tabata #2
Beginner Tabata #7
Beginner Tabata #10
Cooldown with walking, stretching, and rolling

Saturday

Don't let your number of steps drop below Friday's goal.
Play with the kids, dogs, or neighbors; hike just a bit farther. You'll be surprised how the world looks when you're on foot!

This is your off day, no structure needed. Find what you have fun with that includes activity!

Think of it as an active rest day as you transition into your more healthy lifestyle.

THE RESULTS

- Weight loss
- Increased energy from being more active
- Some soreness from working out new muscles
- Few to no feelings of deprivation

Wednesday

Match the steps that you took yesterday!

4 TABATAS

Warm-up
Beginner Tabata #3
Beginner Tabata #5
Beginner Tabata #6
Beginner Tabata #10
Cooldown with walking, stretching, and rolling

Thursday

Take at least 1,000 more steps than you did yesterday.

Repeat Tuesday's cardio. You're starting to get into a routine—be proud of yourself!

5 minutes of casual walking warm-up
2 minutes of speed walking
2 minutes of casual walking
Repeat this for 5 rounds
5-minute cooldown session (includes stretching and foam rolling)

Sunday

4 TABATAS

Warm-up
Beginner Tabata #9
Beginner Tabata #8
Beginner Tabata #2
Beginner Tabata #5
Cooldown with walking, stretching, and rolling

WEEK 2:
Beginner/Intermediate Tabatas + Cutting Back on Sugar

By now, you're on a roll—moving more and feeling positive about everything you accomplished in Week 1. It's crucial to keep this momentum going.

CLEAN

Week 2 objective: *Cut back on added sugar*

- Limit your per-serving added sugar intake to 5 grams—watch out for juices, dried fruit, granola bars, ketchup, and barbecue sauce.
- Be mindful of serving sizes.
- Read all wording on the packaging extra carefully, as it can be misleading.

Add These to Your Grocery List:

100 percent maple syrup	Low-sugar cereal (like Cheerios)	Stevia
Almond butter	Low-sugar ketchup	Your favorite other fruits
Berries	Low-sugar pasta sauces	Your favorite veggies
Club soda	Low-sugar salad dressings	
Dates		
Honey		

Remove These from Your Grocery List:

Artificial sweeteners	Diet and regular soda	Jarred marinades and sauces
Candy	Energy drinks	Tonic water
Chocolate other than dark chocolate	Fruit juice that's not 100 percent natural	White bread products
Cookies		

Try These Breakfasts:
Whole-Wheat Crepes (see page 76)
Easy Yogurt Parfait (see page 78)
Lemon Pancakes with Blueberry Compote (see page 80)
Cheerios with bananas or honey
Apple Cinnamon Oatmeal Pecan Crunch (see page 77)
Smooth Peachiness (see page 106)

Try These Snacks:
Oil-Free Sautéed Almonds (see page 98)
A handful of dates or berries
A KIND bar with 5 grams of added sugar or less
Celery with peanut butter and raisins
Greek yogurt with berries and honey or peanut butter

Try These Lunches:
Apple Cider Salad (see page 82)
Spicy Bahn Mi Wrap (see page 84)
Root Vegetable Tacos (see page 81)
Quinoa Tabouli Salad (see page 86)

Try These Dinners:
Sautéed Brussels Sprouts with Fried Egg (see page 89)
Asian Tuna Steak on a Bed of Sautéed Kale (see page 91)
Chicken Tenders (Traditional Flavor) (see page 87)
Scallop Spinach Salad with Bacon (see page 91)

If You're Craving Dessert:
Frozen grapes
Cookie Dough Hummus (see page 102)
Berry Creme Smoothie (see page 104)

LEAN

Week 2 objective: *Do three or four tabata workouts, each consisting of four to six Beginner Tabatas and/or Intermediate Tabatas.*

- This is when you begin to really challenge yourself physically. Move on to the Intermediate Tabatas as soon as you feel confident with the Beginner Tabatas.
- You can also modify the Beginner Tabatas to make them more challenging. (See page 194 for the five tabata modifications.)

Monday

You should be getting your 10,000 steps every day. This should only rarely be a struggle. Keep at it, as this keeps your frame of mind right!

5 TABATAS

Warm-up
Intermediate Tabata #1
Intermediate Tabata #3
Intermediate Tabata #5
Cardio Tabata #4
Intermediate Tabata #6
Cooldown with walking, stretching, and rolling

Tuesday

10,000 steps. Should be a breeze!
Feeling yesterday's tabatas? The best thing to do with sore muscles is to move. Sitting around will make it worse!

5 minutes of casual walking warm-up
2 minutes of slow jog
1 minute sprint
Repeat the interval for 20 minutes
If needed, walk in between the sprints
5-minute cooldown session (includes stretching and foam rolling)

Friday

10,000 steps. Keep going!

5 TABATAS

Warm-up
Intermediate Tabata #2
Intermediate Tabata #9
Intermediate Tabata #1
Intermediate Tabata #7
Cardio Tabata #5
Cooldown with walking, stretching, and rolling

Saturday

15,000 steps?!
Active rest day. Find what you love and go do it!

BEGINNER/INTERMEDIATE WORKOUT PLAN

If you found the above weekly plan to be challenging, there is nothing wrong with repeating it in week 2. If you need more of a challenge, step up how fast you do the exercises or pick up some heavier weights, all while maintaining correct form. On your cardio days, if the walking portion seems easy, step up how long

Wednesday	**Thursday**
10,000 steps. Keep going!	10,000 steps, as usual
5 TABATAS	Active rest day—just make sure you get your steps
Warm-up	
Intermediate Tabata #8	
Intermediate Tabata #4	
Intermediate Tabata #10	
Intermediate Tabata #6	
Cardio Tabata #3	
Cooldown with walking, stretching, and rolling	

Sunday

10,000 steps

5 TABATAS

Warm-up
Beginner Tabata #2
Beginner Tabata #5
Beginner Tabata #7
Beginner Tabata #6
Beginner Tabata #3
Cooldown with walking, stretching, and rolling

you speed-walk fast or accelerate into jogging. Once you can perform these tabatas without becoming winded, start mixing in Intermediate Tabatas. Week 2 is your plan once you've "graduated" from Beginner Tabatas. Keep in mind, if done with the right modifications, Beginner Tabatas could be on par with an Advanced Tabata workout!

No matter what, don't stop moving during tabatas! If you're doing push-ups, go to your knees. If you're doing squats with jumps, omit the jumping. If you find that jumping lunges are too much, do lunge switches. The most important thing to remember is that these should be hard and you should keep going for all twenty seconds with good form. Even modified exercises will keep your heart rate up.

THE RESULTS

- Continued weight loss
- Continued energy gains from being more active
- Some soreness from working out new muscles
- Increase in muscle tone

WEEK 3:
Intermediate Tabatas + Cutting Back on Sodium

You should be hitting a groove right about now—you've been steadily cleaning up your diet and mastering tabata workouts for two whole weeks. You'll be looking and feeling fantastic. Keep it up!

CLEAN

Week 3 objective: *Cut back on sodium*

- Commit to cutting out processed foods.
- Experiment with herbs, seasonings, and spices.
- Continue to drink lots of water.
- If you're going out to eat, pick a restaurant that makes most of its food from scratch.

Add These to Your Grocery List:

Fresh meat and poultry	Low-sodium string cheese
Low-sodium broths	Low-sodium whole-wheat
Low-sodium salad dressings	wraps and bread products
Low-sodium spices and	Oatmeal
seasonings	

Remove These from Your Grocery List:

Broths	Lunch meats
Cheeses high in sodium	Marinades
Chips and crackers	Most canned goods
Frozen pre-cooked meals	Salad dressings
Gatorade	Soups

Try These Breakfasts:
  Oatmeal with fried egg
  Whole-wheat wrap with eggs and spinach
  Almond flour pancakes
  Avocado toast
  Easy Yogurt Parfait (see page 78)

Try These Snacks:
  Low-sodium string cheese
  Unsalted nuts
  Veggies and low-sodium Greek yogurt dip
  Apple with almond butter
  Brown rice cakes with PB2

Try These Lunches:
  Hummus wrap with veggies
  Kale Salad with Chicken (see page 94)
  Homemade egg salad with whole-wheat toast
  Avocado sandwich with tomato, sprouts, and fat-free mayo

Try These Dinners:
  Seared blackened salmon
  Stir-Fry with Cauliflower Rice (see page 86)
  Chicken Tenders (Italian Blend) (see page 88)
  Asian Tuna Steak on a Bed of Sautéed Kale (see page 91)
  Lemon Pepper Cod (see page 93)

If You're Craving Dessert:
  Peanut Butter Chocolate Protein Brownies
  Almond Butter No-Bake Bar with Berries
  Homemade freezer fruit pops

LEAN

Week 3 objective: *Do three or four tabata workouts, each consisting of four to six Intermediate Tabatas.*

· You can modify the Intermediate Tabatas to make them easier or more challenging. (See page 194 for the five tabata modifications.)

INTERMEDIATE WORKOUT PLAN

As you transition into all Intermediate Tabatas during week 3, your mission remains the same: don't stop moving! Keep challenging your body throughout all eight rounds of each tabata, maintaining proper form the whole time. And by now, you should be able to use the tabata timer like a pro.

THE RESULTS

· Continued weight loss
· Continued energy gains from being more active
· Some soreness from working out new muscles
· Continued increase in muscle tone
· Diminished sugar cravings
· Diminished sodium cravings
· Reduced puffiness

Monday

You should be getting your 10,000 steps every day. This should only rarely be a struggle. Keep at it, as this keeps your frame of mind right!

5 TABATAS

Warm-up
Intermediate Tabata #1
Intermediate Tabata #3
Intermediate Tabata #5
Cardio Tabata #4
Intermediate Tabata #6
Cooldown with walking, stretching, and rolling

Tuesday

10,000 steps—again

Feeling yesterday's tabatas? The best thing to do with sore muscles is to move. Sitting around will make it worse!

5 minutes of casual walking warm-up
2 minutes of slow jog
1 minute sprint
Repeat the interval for 20 minutes
If needed, walk in between the sprints
5-minute cooldown session (includes stretching and foam rolling)

Friday

10,000 steps. Keep going!

5 TABATAS

Warm-up
Intermediate Tabata #2
Intermediate Tabata #9
Intermediate Tabata #1
Intermediate Tabata #7
Cardio Tabata #5
Cooldown with walking, stretching, and rolling

Saturday

15,000 steps?!

Active rest day. Find what you love and go do it!

Wednesday

10,000 steps. Keep going!

5 TABATAS

Warm-up

Intermediate Tabata #8

Intermediate Tabata #4

Intermediate Tabata #10

Intermediate Tabata #6

Cardio Tabata #3

Cooldown with walking, stretching, and rolling

Thursday

10,000 steps

Active rest day—just make sure you get your steps.

Sunday

10,000 steps

5 TABATAS

Warm-up

Intermediate Tabata #2

Intermediate Tabata #5

Intermediate Tabata #7

Intermediate Tabata #6

Intermediate Tabata #3

Cooldown with walking, stretching, and rolling

WEEK 4:
Intermediate/Advanced Tabatas + Cutting Back on Alcohol

Be proud of all you've accomplished so far. At the end of this week, you'll be totally clean and lean. Welcome to the new normal.

CLEAN

Week 4 objective: *Cut back on alcohol, if it's part of your regular diet.*

- Limit yourself to three drinks per week, max.
- Resolve to never drink on a whim.
- Recruit a nondrinking buddy.
- Make it so that you *can't* drink.
- Find tasty nonalcoholic alternatives.
- When you *do* drink, make smart, healthy choices and alternate each one with water.

If you don't want one of the nonalcoholic suggestions from Chapter 4, you can also try one of these with alcohol:
- Vodka soda with a splash of cranberry and a lime
- Tequila on the rocks with a lime
- Light beer (unless there's one *really* good regular beer that you love)
- White wine
- Any of your mocktails with one shot of vodka

I don't want to encourage you to run to the grocery or liquor store and stock up on booze supplies, so there's no new grocery list for this week. I do encourage you to experiment with the healthy nonalcoholic beverage ideas in Chapter 4.

LEAN

Week 4 objective: *Do three or four tabata workouts, each consisting of four to six Intermediate Tabatas and/or Advanced Tabatas*

- When you're ready, you can do all Advanced Tabatas.
- You can also modify the Intermediate Tabatas to make them more challenging. (See page 194 for the five tabata modifications.)

INTERMEDIATE/ADVANCED WORKOUT PLAN

Once the Intermediate Tabatas start to get easy, score that extra challenge by incorporating Advanced Tabatas. Remember that rest days are important, warming up and cooling down are key to reducing injuries, and you can break up the tabatas to fit your schedule.

THE RESULTS

- Continued weight loss
- Continued energy gains from being more active
- Some soreness from working out new muscles
- Continued increase in muscle tone
- Diminished sugar cravings and lower tolerance for sweet foods
- Diminished sodium cravings and lower tolerance for salty foods
- Reduced puffiness
- Diminished alcohol cravings
- Reduced stiffness in joints from all reductions
- Clearer thought processing and better decision making
- A better appreciation for alcoholic beverages you enjoy
- Waking up in a surprisingly good mood each morning
- A heavier wallet
- A true understanding of who your loved ones are—they're the ones who've supported you throughout the past month

Monday

Just because you work out hard doesn't mean you shouldn't get your 10,000 steps every day! An active lifestyle is an all-day thing.

6 TABATAS

Warm-up

Advanced Tabata #3

Advanced Tabata #1

Advanced Tabata #4

Advanced Tabata #2

Advanced Tabata #7

Cardio Tabata #4

Cooldown with stretching and foam rolling

Tuesday

10,000 steps

Soreness abounds today (and possibly tomorrow)! Get your cardio in now with this great routine.

5-minute walking warm-up on treadmill

1.5-minute jog at incline 0

1-minute hill run at incline 7

Repeat this for 20 minutes

5-minute cooldown session with stretching and foam rolling

Note: These hills should be run so that you are super winded. Adjust the speed accordingly! If you don't have a treadmill, find a good, long hill in your area. After a 5-minute warm-up on flat ground, run the hill hard and jog back down to repeat for 20 minutes.

Friday

10,000 steps! The Fitbit has a great option to challenge your friends for a whole weekend. Initiate it now for some friendly competition!

6 TABATAS

Warm-up

Modification #1: all push-ups

Modification #1: all squat jumps

Cardio Tabata #1

Modification #1: all bench dips

Advanced Tabata #6

Advanced Tabata #9

Cooldown with walking, stretching, and foam rolling

Saturday

Your weekend is ripe for a 20,000-step day. Find that perfect hiking spot around town, take your dogs to a park, or walk to a coffee shop you normally drive to. Mix it up!

Day off? Sort of. Keep active in different ways. You're rocking your workouts and deserve a muscle break, but sitting around can make soreness worse. Get out there and explore your town, no matter how large or small it may be.

This is your day to do something different! Cross-train in your favorite activity, whether it's tennis, basketball, soccer, swimming, or rollerblading.

Wednesday

10,000 steps! If your lifestyle allows for more, aim higher. Can you average 15,000 for an entire week?

6 TABATAS

Warm-up
Advanced Tabata #6
Advanced Tabata #8
Advanced Tabata #5
Advanced Tabata #10
Intermediate Tabata #4
Intermediate Tabata #8
Cooldown with walking, stretching, and foam rolling

Thursday

10,000 steps!
Repeat Tuesday's routine for your second cardio session of the week.

Sunday

6 TABATAS!

Warm-up
Intermediate Tabata #1
Intermediate Tabata #3
Modification #1: all burpees
Modification #1: all squats into shoulder presses
Advanced Tabata #2
Advanced Tabata #1
Cooldown with walking, stretching, and foam rolling

IDEAL WEEK OF MEALS

Monday

BREAKFAST
Oatmeal + egg whites topped with fresh berries

SNACK
1 apple + 1 tablespoon almond or peanut butter

LUNCH
Hummus Sandwich (see page 82) + fresh cut fruit salad

SNACK
Banana Blueberry Muffin (see page 99)

DINNER
Zucchini Noodles (see page 93) + tilapia (optional side: Roasted Broccoli with Parmesan Cheese; see page 96)

TIP
Mix in desserts sporadically, when you're *really* craving something sweet, two or three times per week.

Tuesday

BREAKFAST
Avocado Toast with Fried Egg (see page 78)

SNACK
Protein shake or a 4 x 4 smoothie (see page 104)

LUNCH
Kale Salad with Chicken (see page 94), chicken optional

SNACK
1 cup plain Greek yogurt with berries and a touch of honey

DINNER
Chicken Caprese (see page 94) + Mashed Cauliflower (see page 96)

TIP
A strategically made batch of slow-cooker oatmeal can supply more than one meal for you and your family.

Friday

BREAKFAST
Easy Yogurt Parfait (see page 78)

SNACK
Whole-Wheat Banana (see page 100) and/or apple wrap

LUNCH
Chicken Salad (see page 85)

SNACK
Raw veggies + 2 tablespoons hummus

DINNER
Stir-Fry with Cauliflower Rice (see page 86)

SATURDAY

BREAKFAST
Roasted Vegetable Hash with Fried Egg (see page 76)

SNACK
Homemade trail mix

LUNCH
Rice Paper Wraps (see page 83)

SNACK
Almost Butter No-Bake Bar with Berries (see page 101)

DINNER
Kale Salad with Chicken (see page 94)

Wednesday

BREAKFAST
Spinach and egg burrito

SNACK
A KIND bar with 5 grams sugar or less

LUNCH
Root Vegetable Tacos (see page 81)

SNACK
1 serving air-popped popcorn

DINNER
Scallop Spinach Salad with Bacon (see page 91)

TIP
Make note of which meals are especially easy for you to make, and repeat when you're in a pinch.

Thursday

BREAKFAST
Apple Cinnamon Oatmeal Pecan Crunch (see page 77)

SNACK
1 or 2 brown rice cakes with drizzle of honey or almond butter

LUNCH
Spicy Bahn Mi Wrap (see page 84)

SNACK
Light string cheese + a handful of raw almonds

DINNER
Lemon Pancakes with Blueberry Compote (see page 80)

Sunday

BREAKFAST
Whole-Wheat Crepe

SNACK
1 orange or 2 clementines

LUNCH
Quinoa Tabouli Salad

SNACK
Homemade trail mix

DINNER
Traditional or Italian Chicken Tenders (see page 87; optional side: Honey Roasted Butternut Squash, see page 96)

EPILOGUE: NOW WHAT?

If you've reached this page, I trust that you've completed the 4 × 4 Diet's four-week plan. (If not, get out of here!) In just one month, you've found a new normal intake of starches, sugar, sodium, and alcohol. You've toned up your arms, legs, and core through those high-intensity tabata workouts. All that hard work is paying off, and you can see it in how your clothes fit and your body feels. This should excite and motivate you—and excite and motivate your friends and family to join you on this journey. It is exactly why you picked up my book.

Can you believe how different your life was just a month ago? You're now in control of your cravings for starches, sweets, sodium, and booze, and your understanding of sugar as an addiction is hitting home. You're also no longer waking up sore the morning after every workout. Take a moment to close your eyes and really think about how good that feels—and how you earned that feeling. Let's call it the "4 × 4 high."

That incredible feeling is why you have to keep up the clean and lean lifestyle not just for another month or until summer is over, but for the rest of your life. You owe it to yourself to be this healthiest, happiest, absolute best version of you permanently. I've seen it change my clients' lives in the same way—and I'd like to welcome you to the club.

REFERENCES

Chapter 2

http://www.newswise.com/articles/highly-processed-foods-dominate-u-s
-grocery-purchases

http://www.yogajournal.com/article/clean-eating/eat-way-happy-food-mood
-boosting-effects/

http://www.mhhe.com/hper/nutrition/williams/student/appendix_k.pdf

http://www.mayoclinic.org/diseases-conditions/dehydration/basics/symptoms
/con-20030056

http://www.everydayhealth.com/news/unusual-signs-of-dehydration/

http://www.mayoclinic.org/healthy-living/nutrition-and-healthy-eating/in
-depth/water/art-20044256

http://www.npr.org/templates/story/story.php?storyId=106268439

http://www.active.com/fitness/articles/10-things-women-should-know-about
-their-muscles

http://www.ncbi.nlm.nih.gov/pubmed/22890825

http://www.ncbi.nlm.nih.gov/pmc/articles/PMC2996155/

http://www.mayoclinic.org/healthy-living/fitness/in-depth/exercise/art
-20048389?pg=2

http://www.heart.org/HEARTORG/Conditions/More/CardiacRehab
/Frequently-Asked-Questions-About-Physical-Activity_UCM_307388_Article
.jsp

http://www.usatoday.com/story/travel/flights/2014/05/21/airport-walking
-path/9327809/

http://www.ncbi.nlm.nih.gov/pubmed/17414804

Chapter 4

http://www.nlm.nih.gov/medlineplus/ency/article/002469.htm

http://nutritiondata.self.com/facts/vegetables-and-vegetable-products/2770/2

https://www.iom.edu/Reports/2002/Dietary-Reference-Intakes-for-Energy
-Carbohydrate-Fiber-Fat-Fatty-Acids-Cholesterol-Protein-and-Amino-Acids
.aspx

http://www.choosemyplate.gov/food-groups/grains-why.html

http://www.orville.com/healthy-microwave-popcorn-smartpop

http://www.sciencedirect.com/science/article/pii/S0306452205004288

http://www.cdc.gov/nchs/data/databriefs/db122.htm

http://www.cdc.gov/nchs/data/databriefs/db122.htm

http://www.heart.org/HEARTORG/GettingHealthy/NutritionCenter
/HealthyEating/Sugar-101_UCM_306024_Article.jsp

http://www.mayoclinic.org/healthy-living/nutrition-and-healthy-eating/in
-depth/added-sugar/art-20045328

http://www.biomedcentral.com/1471-2458/14/863;

http://www.mayoclinic.org/healthy-living/nutrition-and-healthy-eating/in
-depth/added-sugar/art-20045328?pg=2

http://communitytable.com/324869/erinoprea/8-foods-that-are-surprisingly
-loaded-with-sugar/

http://www.prego.com/sauces/sauces/traditional-italian-sauce/

http://nutritiondata.self.com/facts/dairy-and-egg-products/7578/2

http://www.heart.org/HEARTORG/GettingHealthy/NutritionCenter
/HealthyEating/Sugar-101_UCM_306024_Article.jsp

http://www.foodlabels.com/pdf/RegulatoryGuide-Part4.pdf

http://healthyeating.sfgate.com/roles-sodium-2999.html

http://www.mayoclinic.org/healthy-living/nutrition-and-healthy-eating/in
-depth/sodium/art-20045479

http://www.heart.org/HEARTORG/GettingHealthy/NutritionCenter
/HealthyDietGoals/Reducing-Sodium-in-a-Salty-World_UCM_457519_Article.
jsp

http://www.heart.org/HEARTORG/Conditions/HighBloodPressure
/PreventionTreatmentofHighBloodPressure/Shaking-the-Salt-Habit
_UCM_303241_Article.jsp

http://www.cdc.gov/media/releases/2013/p0903-vs-heart-disease.html

http://www.cdc.gov/dhdsp/vital_signs.htm

http://www.cdc.gov/salt/

http://nutritiondata.self.com/facts/fats-and-oils/7593/2

http://www.npr.org/blogs/thesalt/2012/12/20/167619010/the-paradox-and
-mystery-of-our-taste-for-salt

http://www.webmd.com/a-to-z-guides/potassium-content-of-fruits-vegetables
-and-other-foods-topic-overview

http://nutritiondata.self.com/facts/baked-products/4872/2

http://www.fda.gov/Food/ResourcesForYou/Consumers/ucm315393.htm

http://www.heart.org/HEARTORG/GettingHealthy/NutritionCenter
/HeartSmartShopping/Heart-Check-Food-Certification-Program-Nutrition
-Requirements_UCM_300914_Article.jsp

http://www.health.com/health/gallery/0,,20785388,00.html

http://www.niaaa.nih.gov/alcohol-health/alcohols-effects-body

http://www.nlm.nih.gov/medlineplus/ency/article/000281.htm

http://www.cancer.gov/cancertopics/causes-prevention/risk/alcohol/alcohol
-fact-sheet

http://www.ncbi.nlm.nih.gov/pubmedhealth/PMH0047846

http://www.cancer.org/cancer/news/heavydrinkinglinkedtopancreaticcancer

http://pubs.niaaa.nih.gov/publications/10report/chap04b.pdf

http://www.cdc.gov/alcohol/faqs.htm

Chapter 5

http://almondbreeze.com/?navid=329&pid=508

http://nutritiondata.self.com/facts/dairy-and-egg-products/69/2

http://time.com/3677300/almond-milk-nutrition/

http://nutritiondata.self.com/facts/vegetables-and-vegetable-products/2461/2

http://www.bellplantation.com/nutrition

http://www.jif.com/products/creamy-natural-peanut-butter

http://ndb.nal.usda.gov/ndb/foods/show/2205?fgcd=&manu=&lfacet=&forma
t=&count=&max=35&offset=&sort=&qlookup=avocado

http://nutritiondata.self.com/facts/fruits-and-fruit-juices/1846/2

http://nutritiondata.self.com/facts/breakfast-cereals/1598/2

http://nutritiondata.self.com/facts/dairy-and-egg-products/111/2

http://www.mayoclinic.org/diseases-conditions/high-blood-cholesterol/expert
-answers/cholesterol/faq-20058468

http://nutritiondata.self.com/facts/poultry-products/703/2

http://nutritiondata.self.com/facts/fruits-and-fruit-juices/2064/2

http://nutritiondata.self.com/facts/fruits-and-fruit-juices/1851/2

http://nutritiondata.self.com/facts/fruits-and-fruit-juices/1875/2

http://nutritiondata.self.com/facts/fruits-and-fruit-juices/1848/2

http://nutritiondata.self.com/facts/fruits-and-fruit-juices/2053/2

http://www.ayearofslowcooking.com/2008/11/crockpot-granola-recipe.html

Chapter 6

http://archinte.jamanetwork.com/article.aspx?articleid=1685889

http://nutritiondata.self.com/facts/cereal-grains-and-pasta/5745/2

http://nutritiondata.self.com/facts/cereal-grains-and-pasta/5744/2

http://www.eatingwell.com/healthy_cooking/healthy_cooking_101_basics
_and_techniques/how_to_bake_with_whole_wheat_flour

http://jaha.ahajournals.org/content/4/1/e000993.full

http://nourishedkitchen.com/baking-with-coconut-flour/

http://healthyeating.sfgate.com/health-benefits-oldfashioned-oats-3692.html

http://www.food-allergy.org/spelt.html

http://www.food.com/about/flour-64

http://nutritiondata.self.com/facts/dairy-and-egg-products/78/2

http://www.shape.com/healthy-eating/diet-tips/sugar-wise-how-fruit-stacks

http://healthyeating.sfgate.com/health-benefits-coconut-milk-2031.html

http://nutritiondata.self.com/facts/custom/2098885/2

http://www.webmd.com/food-recipes/how-good-is-soy

http://www.mayoclinic.org/healthy-living/nutrition-and-healthy-eating/expert-answers/butter-vs-margarine/faq-20058152

http://www.fda.gov/Food/ResourcesForYou/Consumers/ucm079609.htm

http://ndb.nal.usda.gov/ndb/foods/show/132?fgcd=&manu=&lfacet=&format=&count=&max=35&offset=&sort=&qlookup=01145

http://www.nytimes.com/2014/03/26/opinion/bittman-butter-is-back.html?_r=0

http://nutritiondata.self.com/facts/custom/1851951/2

http://www.prevention.com/content/which-healthier-butter-or-vegan-buttery-spread

http://earthbalancenatural.com/product/olive-oil-buttery-spread/

http://nutritiondata.self.com/facts/fats-and-oils/7972/2

http://www.olivio.com/products/olive-oil-buttery-spreads-and-sprays/light-olive-oil-buttery-spread/

http://nutritiondata.self.com/facts/sweets/5602/2

http://www.health.com/health/gallery/0,,20424821_4,00.html

http://www.eatingwell.com/nutrition_health/nutrition_news_information/a_healthful_sugar_is_agave_nectar_healthier_than_sugar_o

http://truvia.com/recipes/conversion_chart

Chapter 9

http://journals.lww.com/acsm-msse/Fulltext/1996/10000/Effects_of_moderate_intensity_endurance_and.18.aspx

Chapter 11

http://www.mayoclinic.org/healthy-living/fitness/in-depth/stretching/art-20047931

Chapter 14

http://www.dickssportinggoods.com/product/index.jsp?productId=11783434&

http://www.mayoclinic.org/diseases-conditions/bunions/basics/causes/con-20014535

INDEX